LIPPINCOTT'S
POCKET
NEUROANATOMY

POCKET
NEUROANATOMY

Douglas J. Gould, PhD

LIPPINCOTT'S

POCKET
NEUROANATOMY

Douglas J. Gould, PhD

Professor and Vice Chair

Oakland University William Beaumont School of Medicine

Department of Biomedical Sciences

Rochester, Michigan

 Wolters Kluwer | Lippincott Williams & Wilkins
Health

Philadelphia · Baltimore · New York · London
Buenos Aires · Hong Kong · Sydney · Tokyo

Acquisitions Editor: Crystal Taylor
Product Manager: Lauren Pecarich
Marketing Manager: Joy Fisher Williams
Senior Designer: Stephen Druding
Compositor: Aptara, Inc.

351 West Camden Street
Baltimore, MD 21201

Two Commerce Square
2001 Market Street
Philadelphia, PA 19103

Printed in China

9 8 7 6 5 4 3 2 1

Library of Congress Cataloging-in-Publication Data

Gould, Douglas J.
 Lippincott's pocket neuroanatomy / Douglas J. Gould.
   p. ; cm.
 Pocket neuroanatomy
 Includes index.
 Summary: "Pocket Neuroanatomy, as a part of Lippincott's Pocket Series for the anatomical sciences, is designed to serve time-crunched students. The presentation of neuroanatomy in a table format featuring labeled images efficiently streamlines study and exam preparation for this highly visual and content-rich subject. This pocket-size, quick reference book of neuroanatomical pearls is portable, practical, and necessary; even at this small size, nothing is omitted, and a large number of clinically significant facts, mnemonics, and easy-to-learn concepts are used to complement the tables and inform readers"–Provided by publisher.
 ISBN 978-1-4511-7612-4
 I. Title. II. Title: Pocket neuroanatomy.
 [DNLM: 1. Nervous System–anatomy & histology–Handbooks. WL 39]
 QM451
 611'.8–dc23
                                                                        2013008263

DISCLAIMER

 ᴐ purchase additional copies of this book, call our customer service department at **(800) 638-3030** or orders to **(301) 223-2320**. International customers should call **(301) 223-2300**.

 Lippincott Williams & Wilkins on the Internet: http://www.lww.com. Lippincott Williams & ᴀs customer service representatives are available from 8:30 am to 6:00 pm, EST.

I dedicate this book to my wonderful family—Marie, Maggie, and Lulu—for all of the unconditional love, support, and patience they offer every day of my life.

Health professions curricula around the world are continually evolving: New discoveries, techniques, applications, and content areas compete for increasingly limited time with basic science topics. It is in this context that the foundations established in the basic sciences become increasingly important and relevant for absorbing and applying our ever-expanding knowledge of the human body. As a result of the progressively more crowded curricular landscape, students and instructors are finding new ways to maximize precious contact, preparation, and study time through more efficient, high-yield presentation and study methods.

Pocket Neuroanatomy, as a part of Lippincott's Pocket Series for the anatomical sciences, is designed to serve time-crunched students. The presentation of neuroanatomy in a table format featuring labeled images efficiently streamlines study and exam preparation for this highly visual and content-rich subject. This pocket-size, quick reference book of neuroanatomical pearls is portable, practical, and necessary; even at this small size, nothing is omitted, and a large number of clinically significant facts, mnemonics, and easy-to-learn concepts are used to complement the tables and inform readers.

I am confident that *Pocket Neuroanatomy*, along with other books in the anatomical science Pocket series, will greatly benefit all students attempting to learn clinically relevant foundational concepts in a variety of settings, including all graduate and professional health science programs.

I would like to thank the student and faculty reviewers for their input into this book, which helped create a highly efficient learning and teaching tool. I hope that I have done you justice and created the learning tool that you need.

CONTENTS

Overview of the Nervous System 1

ANATOMY

Orientation

Neuroanatomical terms of orientation are shared with other vertebrates (e.g., fish). However, because we walk upright, when considering the spinal cord, *anterior* is more appropriate than *ventral* and *posterior* more appropriate than *dorsal*. Terminology differs at the **cephalic flexure**, at which point the brain changes orientation with regard to the spinal cord so that humans look forward rather than at the sky (FIG. 1-1).

TERMS OF ORIENTATION	
Brain	**Spinal Cord**
Anterior/rostral	Anterior/ventral
Superior/dorsal	Superior/rostral/cranial
Inferior/ventral	Inferior/caudal
Posterior/caudal	Posterior/dorsal

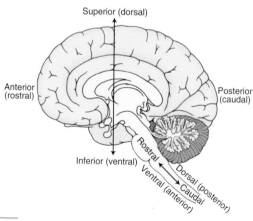

Figure 1-1. Orientation terms.

Central Nervous System

The central nervous system (CNS) is composed of the brain and spinal cord.

DIVISIONS OF THE CENTRAL NERVOUS SYSTEM		
Part	**Division**	**Components**
Brain	Telencephalon	Cerebral hemispheres
		Basal nuclei
	Diencephalon	Epithalamus
		Dorsal thalamus
		Hypothalamus
		Subthalamus
	Brainstem	Midbrain
		Pons
		Medulla
	Cerebellum	Anterior, posterior, and flocculonodular lobes
Spinal cord	One functional unit	Ascending tracts
		Descending tracts
		Interneurons

The paired cerebral hemispheres are separated by the **longitudinal fissure** and **falx cerebri**. They are connected by a large white matter tract, the **corpus callosum**.

Cerebral Hemispheres

The cerebral hemispheres are divided into six lobes (FIGS. 1-2 to 1-4).

Structure	Description	Significance
Frontal lobe	Found within the **anterior cranial fossa** anterior to the **central sulcus** and superior to the **lateral fissure** Composed of: • Precentral gyrus • Superior, middle, and inferior frontal gyri • Gyrus rectus and orbital gyrus	• Contains cortex responsible for higher mental functions (future planning, personality, judgment, social behavior) • Contains primary, supplementary, and premotor cortices • Contains **Broca's area** for motor speech

(continued)

Structure	Description	Significance
Parietal lobe	Found posterior to the central sulcus, superior to the temporal lobe and lateral fissure, and anterior to the occipital lobe Composed of: • Postcentral gyrus • Superior and inferior parietal lobules • Precuneus	• Contains cortex responsible for visual-auditory-spatial sensory integration and orientation • Contains primary and association sensory cortex
Temporal lobe	Found within the **middle cranial fossa** anterior to the occipital lobe and inferior to the lateral fissure Composed of: • Superior, middle, and inferior temporal gyri	• Contains primary and secondary auditory cortex • Contains cortex associated with comprehension of speech: **Wernicke's area**
Occipital lobe	Found within the **posterior cranial fossa** posterior to the parietal lobe Composed of: • Cuneate and lingual gyri	• Contains primary and secondary visual cortex
Limbic lobe	Found on the medial aspect of the cerebral hemispheres Composed of: • Parts of the frontal, parietal, and temporal lobes • Cingulate and parahippocampal gyri	• Functional area associated with memory consolidation and emotion • Functionally divided into the: • Hippocampal formation • Limbic cortex • Amygdala complex

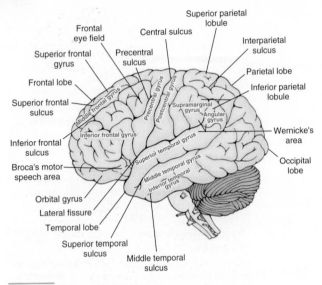

Figure 1-2. Principal gyri and sulci.

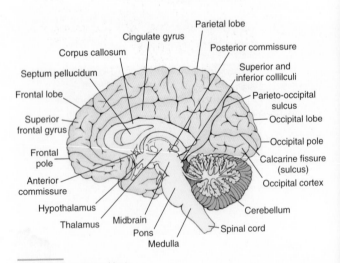

Figure 1-3. Midsagittal brain.

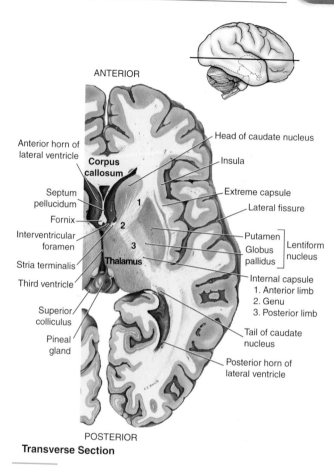

Transverse Section

Figure 1-4. Transverse section through diencephalon.

FIBER PATHWAYS ASSOCIATED WITH THE CEREBRUM

Structure	Description	Significance
Internal capsule	• Funnel-shaped, large white matter tract connecting cerebral cortex with lower centers • Found between the thalamus and basal nuclei • Continuous inferiorly with the **cerebral peduncles** and superiorly with the **corona radiata**	• Divided into five parts: 1. Anterior limb: Connects anterior thalamus-cingulate gyrus and dorso-medial nucleus to prefrontal cortex 2. Posterior limb: Connects motor cortex to ventral anterior and ventral lateral nuclei of thalamus 3. Genu: Blend of fibers from anterior and posterior limbs 4. Sublenticular: Contains **auditory radiations** from medial geniculate nucleus of thalamus to auditory cortex 5. Retrolenticular: Contains **optic radiations** from lateral geniculate nucleus of thalamus to visual cortex
Superior longitudinal fasciculus	• Connects anterior and posterior aspects of each hemisphere • Inferior part connects Broca's and Wernicke's areas—**arcuate fasciculus**	Lesion of the arcuate fasciculus is associated with **conduction aphasia**
Inferior longitudinal fasciculus	Connects the occipital and temporal lobes	Part of the larger occipitotemporal fasciculus
Corpus callosum	Large white matter tract that connects the right and left cerebral hemispheres	Divided into a rostrum, genu, body, and splenium
Anterior commissure	Connects the right and left temporal lobes	Marks the anterior end of the diencephalon
Uncinate fasciculus	Connects the temporal and frontal lobes	Primarily associated with the limbic system, connecting the temporal lobe limbic structures with the orbitofrontal cortex
Cingulum	Large white matter pathway that connects parts of the limbic cortex	Found within the cingulate and parahippocampal gyri

Additional Concepts

White matter fiber pathways that connect cortical areas within a hemisphere are known as association tracts or bundles; those connecting the hemispheres are commissural.

Basal Nuclei

Subcortical nuclei of the telencephalon that are associated with the motor system.

Structure	Description	Significance
Caudate	• Together with the putamen forms the **neostriatum** • More medial part of the corpus striatum	• Extensive connections with cerebral association cortex (i.e., prefrontal cortex) • Cognitive aspects of movement
Putamen	• Together with the caudate forms the **neostriatum** • More lateral part of the corpus striatum	• Forms the outer part of the **lentiform nucleus** along with the globus pallidus • The majority of the motor-oriented cerebral input into the basal nuclei is to the putamen
Globus pallidus	• Located medial to the putamen • Divided into external and internal parts	• External part receives input from the striatum and outputs primarily to the subthalamic nucleus • Internal part receives afferents from subthalamic nucleus and striatum and projects to the thalamus
Subthalamic nucleus	• Part of the diencephalon • Key component of the **indirect pathway** through the system	• Receives afferents from the external segment of the globus pallidus • Projects excitatory efferents to the internal segment of the globus pallidus

Additional Concepts

BASAL GANGLIA

The basal nuclei are often referred to as the basal ganglia. However, because they are accumulations of neuronal cell bodies found within the CNS, *basal nuclei* is the more appropriate term.

The term *neostriatum* is often shortened to *striatum* in common usage.

TERMINOLOGY ASSOCIATED WITH THE BASAL NUCLEI

Term	Structures Included
Corpus striatum	Caudate, putamen, and globus pallidus
Neostriatum or striatum	Caudate and putamen
Pallidum	Globus pallidus (both parts)
Lentiform or lenticular nucleus	Putamen and globus pallidus

FIBER PATHWAYS ASSOCIATED WITH THE BASAL NUCLEI

Structure	Description	Significance
Ansa lenticularis	• Efferent fiber pathway originating from the internal segment of globus pallidus	Loops around the **internal capsule** to join the **thalamic fasciculus**
Lenticular fasciculus	• Conveys inhibitory influence to the ventral lateral nucleus of the thalamus	Passes through the internal capsule to join the thalamic fasciculus
Thalamic fasciculus	Fiber pathway containing the fibers of the combined ansa lenticularis and lenticular fasciculus, as well as projections from the cerebellum	• Fibers from basal nuclei synapse on ventral lateral nucleus of the thalamus • Fibers from cerebellum synapse on ventral anterior nucleus of the thalamus
Nigrostriatal pathway	Fiber pathway projecting from the **substantia nigra pars compacta** to the striatum	Dopamine into the striatum from the substantia nigra modifies activity through the basal nuclei
Striatonigral pathway	Fiber pathway projecting from the striatum to the substantia nigra	Efferents from the striatum to substantia nigra release γ-aminobutyric acid (GABA) to decrease output from the substantia nigra

Additional Concepts

Two classically described pathways through the basal nuclei are commonly presented (FIG. 1-5), although it should be noted that the interconnections of the nuclei and associated structures are more numerous and complex than is possible to present here.

Disinhibition: When the nucleus responsible for inhibiting the activity of a second inhibitory nucleus, the end result is activity, or in this case, disinhibition.

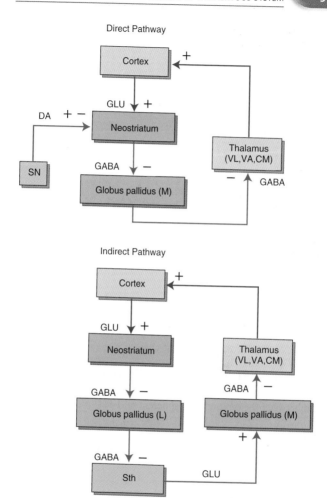

Figure 1-5. Direct and indirect pathways.

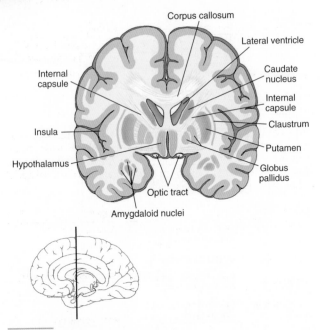

Figure 1-6. Frontal section through diencephalon.

Diencephalon

The diencephalon is located immediately cranial to the brainstem and between the cerebral hemispheres (FIG. 1-6).

Structure	Description	Significance
(Dorsal) thalamus	• Extends anteriorly to the anterior commissure, inferiorly to the **hypothalamic sulcus,** and posteriorly to the posterior commissure • Thalami are separated by the third ventricle	All sensory information, except olfaction, connects with the thalamus as it passes to the cerebral cortex
Hypothalamus	Extends superiorly to the hypothalamic sulcus	Coordinates drive-related behaviors through control of the autonomic nervous system and maintains homeostasis

(continued)

Structure	Description	Significance
Epithalamus	Posterior-most part of the diencephalon	Primary components are the **pineal gland** and **habenula**
Subthalamus	Primary component is the subthalamic nucleus	Functionally related to the basal nuclei

Thalamus (Dorsal)

The largest part of the diencephalon, the dorsal thalamus—or, more commonly, the thalamus—consists of two large ovoid groups of nuclei, typically interconnected by an interthalamic adhesion (FIG. 1-7). The thalami receive most of the input from the basal nuclei and all sensory input except for olfaction.

Nucleus	Input	Output
Lateral dorsal	Mamillothalamic tract	Cingulate gyrus
Lateral posterior	Parietal cortex (areas 1 and 5)	
Ventral anterior	Basal nuclei	
Ventral lateral	Basal nuclei, cerebellum and red nucleus	Motor cortex (areas 4 and 6)
Ventral posterior lateral	Spinothalamic tracts and medial lemniscus	Sensory cortex (areas 3, 1 and 2)
Ventral posterior medial	Trigeminothalamic tracts, taste (solitary nucleus)	
Dorsomedial	Prefrontal and orbital cortex and intralaminar nuclei	Prefrontal and orbital cortex, amygdala, and temporal cortex
Midline	Motor cortex (area 4) and globus pallidus	Motor cortex (area 4), striatum, and diffuse to entire cortex
Anterior	Hypothalamus via mamillo-thalamic tract and hippocampus via fornix	Cingulate gyrus
Pulvinar	Association cortex of the parietal, occipital, and temporal lobes; medial and lateral geniculate nuclei; and superior colliculus	Association cortex of parietal, occipital, and temporal lobes
Medial geniculate	Cochlear nerve > Inferior colliculus	Primary auditory cortex (areas 41 and 42)
Lateral geniculate	Retina > Optic tract	Primary visual cortex (area 17) via the optic radiations
Reticular nucleus	All thalamic nuclei	

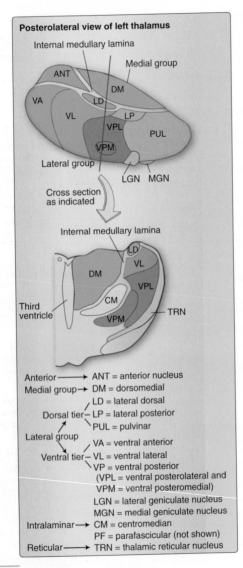

Posterolateral view of left thalamus

Internal medullary lamina

Medial group

ANT

DM

VA

LD

VL

LP

VPL

VPM

PUL

Lateral group

LGN   MGN

Cross section as indicated

Internal medullary lamina

LD

VL

DM

VPL

Third ventricle

CM

VPM

TRN

| Anterior | → | ANT = anterior nucleus |
| Medial group | → | DM = dorsomedial |

Dorsal tier —
- LD = lateral dorsal
- LP = lateral posterior
- PUL = pulvinar

Lateral group ↗

Ventral tier —
- VA = ventral anterior
- VL = ventral lateral
- VP = ventral posterior
  (VPL = ventral posterolateral and
  VPM = ventral posteromedial)

LGN = lateral geniculate nucleus
MGN = medial geniculate nucleus

Intralaminar → CM = centromedian
PF = parafascicular (not shown)

Reticular → TRN = thalamic reticular nucleus

Figure 1-7. The thalamus.

Hypothalamus

The hypothalamus is the inferior-most portion of the diencephalon. It functions with the endocrine system to maintain homeostasis and governs the activities of the autonomic nervous system. It is divided into a series of regions, each of which contain a variety of nuclei (Fig. 1-8). It is also divided into medial and lateral zones.

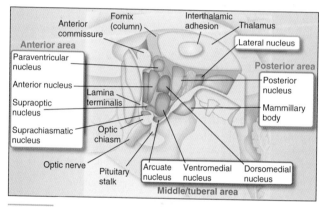

Figure 1-8. The hypothalamic nuclei.

Region	Zone	Nuclei	Function
Anterior	Medial	Preoptic	Contains **sexually dimorphic nucleus**; regulates release of gonadotropic hormones; parasympathetic activity
		Supraoptic	Secretes oxytocin and vasopressin
		Paraventricular	Secretes oxytocin and vasopressin (magnocellular part); secretes corticotropin-releasing hormone (parvocellular part)
		Anterior	Involved in thermoregulation; destruction causes hypothermia; role in sleep regulation
		Suprachiasmatic	Plays a role in circadian rhythms
	Lateral	Lateral nuclei	Initiates eating and drinking

(continued)

Region	Zone	Nuclei	Function
Middle or Tuberal	Medial	Dorsomedial	Plays a role in circadian rhythms, feeding, and emotions
		Ventromedial	Satiety center
		Arcuate	Secrete growth hormone–releasing hormone
	Lateral	Lateral nuclei	Initiates eating and drinking
Posterior	Medial	Mammillary bodies	Memory consolidation
		Posterior nucleus	Heat conservation center, arousal, wakefulness
	Lateral	Lateral nuclei	Initiates eating and drinking

Additional Concepts

In general terms, the anterior and medial aspects of the hypothalamus have a more "parasympathetic" role, and the posterior and lateral aspects have a more "sympathetic" function.

There exist functional centers in the hypothalamus:

1. Temperature regulation
   a. Anterior hypothalamus lesion = Hyperthermia
   b. Posterior hypothalamus lesion = Hypothermia
2. Food intake
   a. Ventromedial nucleus lesion = Hyperphagia
   b. Lateral hypothalamus lesion = Hypophagia
3. Sleep–wake cycle
   a. Anterior hypothalamus lesion = Insomnia
   b. Posterior hypothalamus lesion = Hypersomnia
4. Emotions: lesion of the ventromedial nucleus = Rage
5. Water balance: Lesion of the anterior hypothalamus = Diabetes insipidus

Brainstem

The brainstem (FIG. 1-9) is the phylogenetically oldest part of the brain. Cranially, it is continuous with the diencephalon, and caudally it is continuous with the spinal cord. In addition to providing an important conduit function, it contains circuitry for respiratory and cardiac reflex activity.

Structure	Description	Significance
Midbrain (mesencephalon)	• Superior-most part of brainstem • Possesses a **tectum** composed of the **superior** and **inferior colliculi** • Anterior surface has **cerebral peduncles**	• Contains the **cerebral aqueduct** • Gives rise to the **trochlear nerve** (cranial nerve [CN] IV)
Pons	• Found between the midbrain and medulla • Located anterior to the cerebellum, to which it is connected by **cerebellar peduncles**	• Gives rise to the **trigeminal** (CN V), **abducent** (CN VI), **facial** (CN VII), and **vestibulocochlear** (CN VIII) nerves
Medulla	• Inferiormost part of brainstem • Continuous inferiorly with spinal cord at **foramen magnum** • Anterior surface has **pyramids**	• Gives rise to the **glossopharyngeal** (CN IX), **vagal** (CN X), and **hypoglossal** (CN XII) nerves

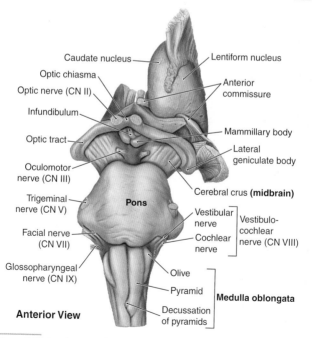

Figure 1-9. Anterior view of brainstem. (*continued*)

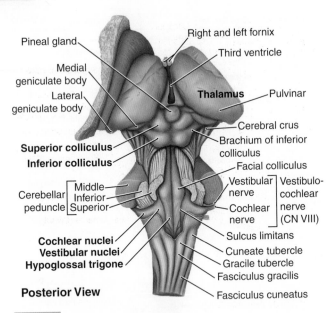

Figure 1-9. (continued) Posterior view of brainstem.

Cerebellum

The cerebellum is involved in the planning, coordination, and modification of motor activities (FIG. 1-10).

Structure	Description	Significance
Anterior-to-posterior divisions	• Anterior • Posterior • Flocculonodular	• Anterior is separated from posterior by a **primary fissure** • Posterior is separated from flocculonodular by a **posterolateral fissure**
Lateral-to-medial divisions	• Lateral hemisphere • Medial (paravermal) hemisphere • Vermis	Lateral-to-medial divisions are based on functional connections
Cerebellar peduncles	• Superior • Middle • Inferior	Connect the cerebellum to the brainstem, mainly the pons

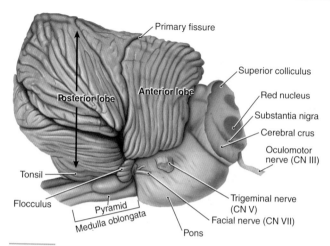

Figure 1-10. Lateral view of cerebellum and brainstem.

Peripheral Nervous System

The peripheral nervous system (PNS) is composed of all parts of the nervous system that are not brain or spinal cord, including the cranial and spinal nerves, plexuses, and receptors.

Peripheral Receptors

Nervous system receptors (FIG. 1-11) may be classified by function, axon diameter or conduction velocity or fiber type, morphology or structure, or level of adaptation.

Type of Mechanoreceptor	Structure	Sensory Modality	Fiber Type	Adaptation
Free nerve endings	Unencapsulated: No connective tissue covering on end of nerve fibers	Pain and temperature	A-δ C (unmyelinated)	Variable
Merkel's disc		Crude touch	A-β or type II	Slow

(continued)

Type of Mechanoreceptor	Structure	Sensory Modality	Fiber Type	Adaptation
Pacinian corpuscle	Encapsulated: End of nerve fibers enclosed in connective tissue, which assists in receptor function	Pressure and vibration		Very fast
Meissner's corpuscle		Fine touch	A-β or type II	Fast
Ruffini corpuscle		Tension and stretch		
Muscle spindle		Muscle stretch	A-α or type Ia A-β or type II	Slow
Golgi tendon organ		Muscle tension	A-α or type Ib	

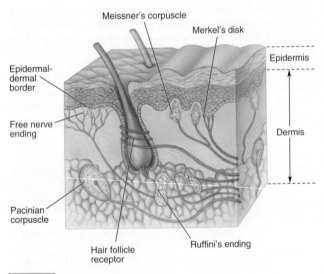

Figure 1-11. Peripheral receptors in the skin.

			NERVE FIBERS	
Alphabetical Class	Numerical Class	Myelinated or Unmyelinated	Conduction Velocity (M/Sec)	Innervate
A-α	Ia	Myelinated	80–120	Annulospiral endings of muscle spindles
	Ib			Golgi tendon organs
A-β	II		35–75	Flower-spray endings from muscle spindles
A-δ	III		5–30	Fibers conducting crude touch, pain, and temperature
C	IV	Unmyelinated	0.5–2	Fibers conducting pain and temperature

Additional Concepts

Typically, the alphabetical classification system is used for motor fibers, and the numerical is used for sensory fibers. There are many exceptions; for instance, "slow pain" is carried on C fibers, not typically referred to as type IV fibers.

Peripheral Nerves

A nerve is a collection of axons bound together by connective tissue that serves to transmit electrical signals between the CNS and the periphery (FIG. 1-12).

Structure	Description	Significance
Cranial nerve	• Olfactory (CN I): Sensory only	• CN I: Special sense of smell
	• Optic (CN II): Sensory only	• CN II: Special sense of vision
	• Oculomotor (CN III): Motor only	• CN III: Motor to four of six extraocular muscles; parasympathetic to sphincter pupillae and ciliaris, and superior tarsal
	• Trochlear (CN IV): Motor only	• CN IV: Motor to superior oblique

(continued)

Structure	Description	Significance
Cranial nerve	• Trigeminal (CN V): Both sensory and motor	• CN V: Sensory to face; motor to eight muscles, including the muscles of mastication
	• Abducens (CN VI): Motor only	• CN VI: Motor to lateral rectus
	• Facial (CN VII): Both sensory and motor	• CN VII: Motor to muscles of facial expression; sensory to external ear; parasympathetic to submandibular and sublingual salivary glands and lacrimal gland; special sense of taste to anterior 2/3 of tongue
	• Vestibulocochlear (CN VIII): Sensory only	• CN VIII: Special sense of hearing and equilibrium
	• Glossopharyngeal (CN IX): Both sensory and motor	• CN IX: Motor to stylopharyngeus; parasympathetic to parotid gland; sensory to pharynx and middle ear; special sense of taste to posterior 1/3 of tongue
	• Vagus (CN X): Both sensory and motor	• CN X: Motor to palate, larynx, and pharynx; parasympathetic to thorax and abdomen; sensory to external ear
	• Spinal accessory (CN XI): motor only	• CN XI: Motor to sternocleidomastoid and trapezius
	• Hypoglossal (CN XII): Motor only	• CN XII: Motor to tongue musculature

Spinal nerve	• 31 pairs
	• Formed by the merging of anterior and posterior roots
	• Terminates as anterior and posterior primary rami
		• Divided into:
		  • 8 cervical spinal nerve pairs (C1–C8)
		  • 12 thoracic pairs (T1–T12)
		  • 5 lumbar pairs (L1–L5)
		  • 5 sacral pairs (S1–S5)
		  • 1 coccygeal pair
		• May contain postganglionic sympathetic, somatic motor, and sensory fibers

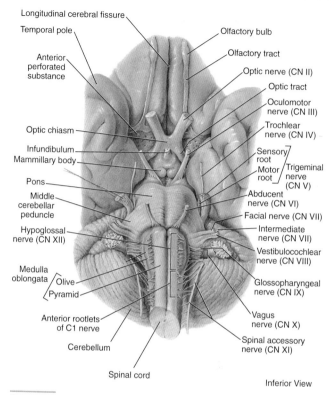

Figure 1-12. Cranial nerves on base of brain.

Additional Concepts

CN I is really a loose grouping of fibers from bipolar cells suspended in the upper aspect of the nasal cavity: the fila olfactoria. CN XI originates from the posterior aspect of the anterior horn in the cervical spinal cord and is therefore not actually a cranial nerve.

Anterior and posterior roots (rootlets) join to form the **spinal nerve**. The actual spinal nerve is a very short structure about 1 cm in length, although the term is often used loosely to describe the nerves of the PNS. The spinal nerve terminates by dividing into an **anterior** and **posterior ramus**. Somatic plexuses, such as the **cervical, brachial,** and **lumbosacral,** are formed only by **anterior rami; posterior rami** remain segmental.

Each pair of spinal nerves (or spinal cord segment) supplies a strip of skin with sensory innervation: a **dermatome**. This often differs from the **pattern of cutaneous innervation**, which is the area of skin supplied with sensory innervation by an individual peripheral nerve. This is a result of peripheral nerves emerging from **plexuses**, where anterior rami join and exchange fibers from different spinal cord levels. In the trunk, there is no plexus formation, and the pattern of cutaneous innervation and the dermatome are the same.

MNEMONIC

On old Olympus' towering tops; a fin and German viewed some hops.

This phrase corresponds to the names of cranial nerves.

- **O**lfactory (CN I)
- **O**ptic (CN II)
- **O**culomotor (CN III)
- **T**rochlear (CN IV)
- **T**rigeminal (CN V)
- **A**bducens (CN VI)
- **F**acial (CN VII)
- **V**estibulocochlear (CN VIII), formerly known as the **a**uditory nerve
- **G**lossopharyngeal (CN IX)
- **V**agus (CN X)
- **S**pinal accessory (CN XI)
- **H**ypoglossal (CN XII)

Some say marry money, but my brother says big brains matter more.

This phrase corresponds to the functions of cranial nerves.

- Olfactory (CN I): **S**ensory
- Optic (CN II): **S**ensory
- Oculomotor (CN III): **M**otor
- Trochlear (CN IV): **M**otor
- Trigeminal (CN V): **B**oth sensory and motor
- Abducens (CN VI): **M**otor
- Facial (CN VII): **B**oth sensory and motor
- Vestibulocochlear (CN VIII): **S**ensory

- Glossopharyngeal (CN IX): **B**oth sensory and motor
- Vagus (CN X): **B**oth sensory and motor
- Spinal Accessory (CN XI): **M**otor
- Hypoglossal (CN XII): **M**otor

Spinal Cord

The spinal cord extends from the foramen magnum, where it is continuous with the medulla, to a tapering end called the **medullary cone**, at the L1 to L2 vertebral level (FIG. 1-13). It serves as a reflex center and conduction pathway, connecting the brain to the periphery. It gives rise to 31 pairs of spinal nerves.

Feature	Description	Significance
Cervical enlargement	Enlarged part of spinal cord between C4 and T1	Gives rise to anterior rami that form the **brachial plexus**; innervates upper limbs
Lumbar enlargement	Enlarged part of spinal cord between L1 and S3	Gives rise to anterior rami that form the **lumbosacral plexus**; innervates lower limbs
Medullary cone	Tapered, inferior end of spinal cord	• Located at L1–L2 vertebral level • Nerve roots near conus contribute to **cauda equina**
Cauda equina	Collection of anterior and posterior roots from inferior aspect of spinal cord	Located in the **lumbar cistern**; a continuation of the subarachnoid space in the **dural sac** caudal to the medullary cone
Gray matter	Located on the inside of the spinal cord, deep to the white matter	Divided into posterior, lateral (between T1 and L2), and anterior horns
White matter	Located on the outside of the spinal cord, external to the gray matter	Divided into anterior, lateral, and posterior funiculi; contains ascending and descending fiber tracts

DEVELOPMENT

The nervous system begins to form in the third week of development. The first evidence of the developing nervous system is a thickening of the ectoderm of the trilaminar embryo, the **neural plate** (FIG. 1-14).

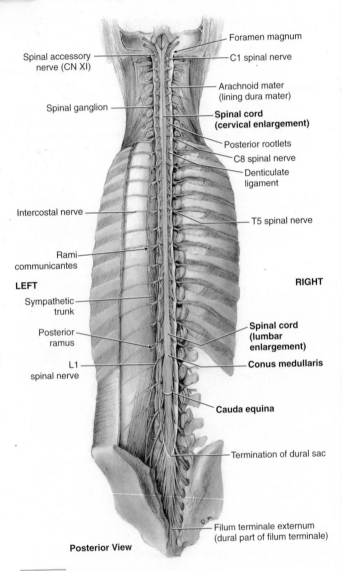

Figure 1-13. The spinal cord.

Day First Appears	Structure	Significance
18	Neural plate	Thickening of ectoderm between **primitive node** and **oropharyngeal membrane**
20	Neural groove Neural fold	Continued thickening of the neural plate on its periphery forms a midline neural groove, with the thickened neural folds along the side of the groove
22	Neural tube	• Neural folds join in the midline to form the neural tube; fusion of the folds proceeds cranially and caudally, eventually leaving a **cranial** and **caudal neuropore** • Neural tube separates from surface ectoderm to lie between it and the **notochord** • Cranial part of neural tube forms the brain; caudal portion forms spinal cord; lumen of the tube forms central canal of spinal cord and ventricular system of brain
	Cranial neuropore	Closes on ~day 25; forms **lamina terminalis** in adult
	Caudal neuropore	Closes on ~day 27

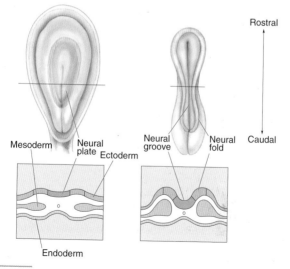

Figure 1-14. Dorsum of embryo. (*continued*)

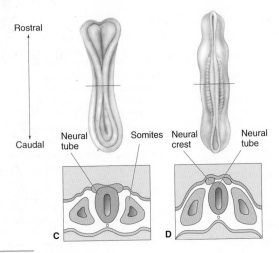

Figure 1-14. (*continued*)

Clinical Significance

Failure of the cranial neuropore to close may cause **anencephaly,** a serious birth defect in which the brain and cranial vault fail to develop. Failure of the caudal neuropore to close may lead to **spinal bifida,** which includes the following variants (presented in order of severity):

- Occulta: Vertebral arch defect only
- Cystica, which has two forms:
  - Meningocele: Meninges project through vertebral arch defect, forming a cerebrospinal fluid (CSF)–filled cyst
  - Meningomyelocele: Spinal cord tissue projects through vertebral arch defect into CSF-filled meningeal cyst
- Myeloschisis: Open neural tube

Neural Crest

The neural crest is a migratory population of pluripotent cells that disassociate during formation of the neural tube (FIG. 1-15). Neural crest cells migrate throughout the body to form a multitude of structures in adults.

Structure	Significance
Leptomeninges	Forms the pia mater and arachnoid
Cells of the autonomic ganglia	Postganglionic sympathetic and parasympathetic cell bodies
Cells of the spinal and cranial nerve ganglia	First-order sensory cell bodies
Schwann cells	Form myelin in the peripheral nervous system
Chromaffin cells	Neuroendocrine cells found in the adrenal medulla
Melanocytes	Pigment-producing cells of the epidermis
Pharyngeal arch skeleton	Skeletal and connective tissue components of the pharyngeal arches
Aorticopulmonary septum	Connective tissue septum that divides the aorta and pulmonary trunk in the heart
Odontoblasts	Cells that form dentin in the teeth
Parafollicular cells	Calcitonin-producing cells of the thyroid gland

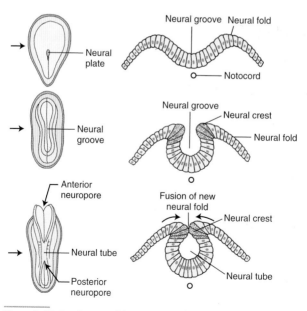

Figure 1-15. Development of the central nervous system.

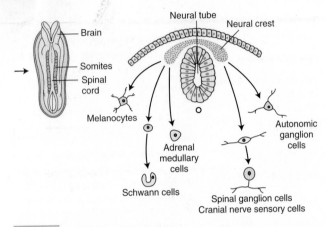

Figure 1-15. Development of the central nervous system.

Clinical Significance

Because neural crest cells migrate so widely throughout the body and are responsible for the appropriate formation of so many structures, disruption of their migration often causes debilitating syndromes such as Treacher Collins and Pierre Robin syndrome, which may affect the face, heart, metabolism, and nervous system.

Neural Tube

During the fourth week of gestation, the neural tube expands and dilates to form vesicles (Fig. 1-16). The lumen of the tube forms the ventricular system of the brain.

Primary Vesicle	Secondary Vesicle	Adult Structure	Ventricular System
Prosencephalon (forebrain)	Telencephalon	Cerebral hemispheres Olfactory bulbs	Lateral (two) ventricles
	Diencephalon	Thalami	Third ventricle
Mesencephalon (midbrain)	Mesencephalon	Midbrain	Cerebral aqueduct

(continued)

Primary Vesicle	Secondary Vesicle	Adult Structure	Ventricular System
	Cephalic Flexure		
Rhombencephalon (hindbrain)	Metencephalon	Pons	Fourth ventricle
		Cerebellum	
	Myelencephalon	Medulla	
	Cervical Flexure		
	Developing Spinal Cord		

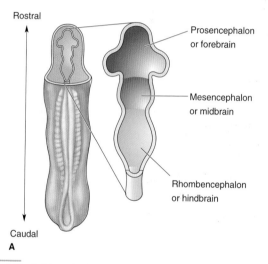

Figure 1-16. **A.** Primary brain vesicles. (*continued*)

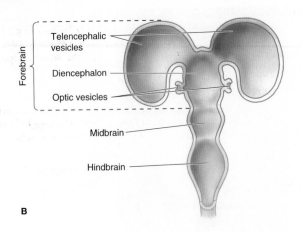

B

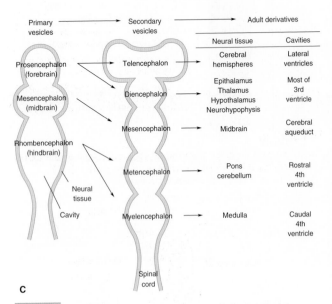

C

Figure 1-16. (*continued*) **B.** Secondary brain vesicles. **C.** Derivatives of the vesicles.

Additional Concepts

Thickenings of the neural ectoderm give rise to (1) **olfactory plac-odes**, which form CN I and induce formation of the **olfactory bulbs**, and (2) **otic placodes**, which form CN VIII and the sensory appa-ratuses of the inner ear.

Clinical Significance

Hydrocephalus is a dilation of the developing ventricles caused by excessive CSF, typically resulting from failure (blockage) of the ventricular drainage system to remove CSF and move it into the circulation.

Neural Tube Wall

The neural tube wall is divided into three layers.

Layer	Location	Significance
Neuroepithelium (ventricular)	Innermost: Adjacent to the lumen of tube	Formed of **ependymal cells** that line central canal and ventricles
Mantle (interme-diate)	Middle layer	Formed of neurons and glia; gives rise to gray matter
Marginal	Outermost	Contains nerve fibers from neurons and glia; gives rise to white matter

Spinal Cord

The spinal cord develops from the neural tube, caudal to the fourth pair of somites. It is divided transversely into plates (FIG. 1-17).

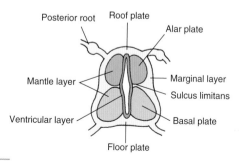

Figure 1-17. Cross-section through developing spinal cord.

Plate	Position	Adult Structures
Alar	Posterior/lateral	Posterior horns: Sensory
	Sulcus Limitans: Separates alar from basal plate	
Basal	Anterior/lateral	Anterior horns: Motor
Roof	Posterior	Posterior covering of central canal
Floor	Anterior	Anterior white commissure

Additional Concepts

The sulcus limitans is visible in the floor of the fourth ventricle in the adult brainstem and is a useful guide for separating motor and sensory nuclei.

In an infant, the spinal cord extends the length of the vertebral canal; growth of the vertebral canal outpaces that of the spinal cord such that in an adult, the spinal cord only extends to the L1 to L2 vertebral level.

Clinical Significance

The dural sac continues to the inferiormost aspect of the vertebral canal. It is filled with the cauda equina, filum terminale, and CSF; thus, because the spinal cord ends at L1 to L2, the dural sac is an excellent place from which to remove CSF as is done in a spinal tap.

NEUROHISTOLOGY

The cells of the nervous system—neurons and glia—are derived from neuroectoderm (FIGS. 1-18 and 1-19).

Cell Type	General Characteristics	Identifying Characteristics
Neuron	• Generally not capable of dividing • Capable of sending and receiving electrochemical signals • Composed of cell body, dendrites, and an axon	• **Multipolar:** Most common; one axon and multiple dendrites; motor neurons and interneurons • **Bipolar:** Sensory only; ganglia of CN VIII, retina, and olfactory epithelium

Cell Type	General Characteristics	Identifying Characteristics
	• Motor neurons conduct signals to effector organs; sensory neurons receive signals from receptors; interneurons (internuncial) connect motor and sensory neurons and have an integrative function	• **Pseudounipolar:** Sensory; sensory ganglia of cranial nerves and spinal ganglia; mesencephalic nucleus

Astrocyte	• Most common cell-type in CNS
	• Function in/as:
	  • Blood–brain barrier
	  • Ion buffer
	  • Glial scar
	  • Structural support
	  • Glycogen reserve
	  • Metabolic support
	  • Neurotransmitter sink
	  • Synaptic modifier
		• **Fibrous:** Found in white matter
		• **Protoplasmic:** Found in gray matter
		• **Radial:** Role in guiding neuronal migration during development

Microglia	• Monocytic origin • Serve as macrophages • migratory	• **Activated:** Phagocytic role • **Resting:** Inactive form
Oligodendrocyte	Myelin-forming cells of CNS; one oligodendrocyte may myelinate parts of several axons	• **Satellite cells:** Found in gray matter • **Interfascicular:** Found in white matter
Ependymal	Epithelial cells that line central canal and ventricles	Are the epithelial component of the **choroid plexus**, which makes CSF
Schwann	Myelin-forming cells of PNS; one Schwann cell myelinates one internode of one axon	Invest and provide support for unmyelinated axons

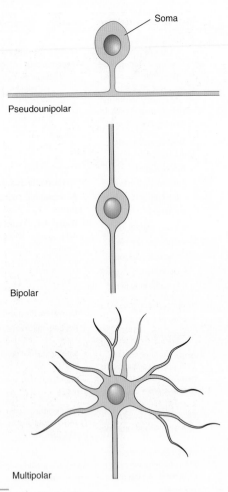

Figure 1-18. Classification of neurons.

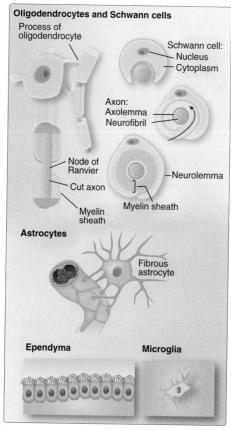

Figure 1-19. Glia.

Additional Concepts

Myelin is an electrically insulating wrapping of nerve fibers that forms the myelin sheath. The nerve fibers are wrapped in segments called internodes, with gaps in between called the nodes of Ranvier (FIG. 1-20). The action potential is able to "skip" from node to node in a process called saltatory conduction, thus speeding the signal towards the synapse.

PARTS OF A NEURON (FIG. 1-20)		
Part	Structure	Significance
Cell body (soma)	• Large nucleus with **Nissl substance** (rough endoplasmic reticulum (rER)) • Large nucleolus • Lots of mitochondria	• Significant rER is evidence of large protein synthesis role • Cytoskeletal elements composed of neurofilaments, microfilaments and microtubules; for vesicle transport, axonal growth and structure
Axon	• Single • May be myelinated or unmyelinated • Active transport: **Anterograde** (away from soma), **Retrograde** (toward soma)	
Dendrite(s)	May range from one to multiple	• Conduct impulses towards the cell body • May possess **dendritic spines**: Site of synaptic contact

Additional Concepts

An individual nerve fiber and myelin sheath (if present) is wrapped in a layer of connective tissue: the **endoneurium**; the **perineurium** wraps multiple fibers together in a **fascicle**. Fascicles and small blood vessels are wrapped in **epineurium** to form a peripheral nerve.

Clinical Significance

Axons in the PNS are capable of regeneration if the part of the axon distal to the injury is still intact and the endoneurial sheath is still patent.

MENINGES

The meninges protect and support the brain and spinal cord (FIG. 1-21). From outside to in, the meninges are the dura mater, arachnoid, and pia mater (FIG. 1-22).

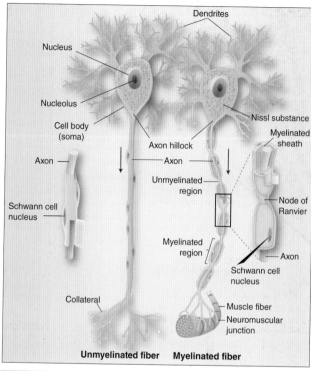

Figure 1-20. The neuron.

MENINGES AND SPACES AROUND THE BRAIN

Layer (from outside to in)	Description	Significance
	Skull	
Epidural space	• Potential space • Contains meningeal arteries and veins	Site of epidural hematoma; typically results from trauma to a meningeal artery

(continued)

Layer (from outside to in)	Description	Significance
Dura mater	• Tough, inflexible outer layer • Adherent to inside of cranial vault • Supplied with blood by meningeal arteries	• Separates into two layers to form **dural septa** in several locations • Sensitive to pain (e.g., from stretching); supratentorial dura is innervated by CN V; infratentorial dura is innervated by CN X
Subdural space	Potential space	Site of subdural hematoma; typically results from damage to cranial (bridging) veins
Arachnoid mater	• Delicate layer; adherent to dura by CSF pressure and **dural border cells** • Part of the **leptomeninges** with the pia mater	• Avascular • Lines the dura mater • Evaginations of arachnoid through the dura enter the **superior sagittal sinus** via **arachnoid villi** to allow CSF to move from subarachnoid space to venous system
Subarachnoid space	• CSF-filled space between the arachnoid and pia • Expanded in several areas where the arachnoid bridges over surface irregularities of the brain to form CSF-filled **subarachnoid cisterns** (i.e., **cisterna magna**)	• Site of subarachnoid hemorrhage; could be either a cerebral artery or vein • Spanned by **arachnoid trabeculae**, which help stabilize the brain
Pia mater	• Part of the leptomeninges with the arachnoid mater • Adherent to surface of brain	• Highly vascularized membrane • Extends along proximal ends of blood vessels as **perivascular space**

Brain

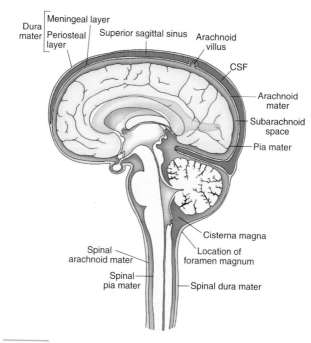

Figure 1-21. The meninges.

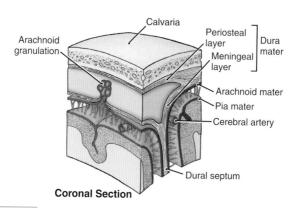

Figure 1-22. The meninges (magnified view).

Clinical Significance

Inflammation of the meninges: Meningitis may be viral, bacterial, or caused by some microorganism. It is considered severe owing to its ability to spread quickly around the CNS and because of the proximity of the meninges to the brain and spinal cord.

Dural Folds and Sinuses

In several areas in the cranial vault, the dura mater separates into two distinct layers: a **periosteal layer** that lines the skull and a **meningeal layer** that forms **dural septa** that extend into the cranial cavity between parts of the brain for support (FIG. 1-23). In the attached edge of each of the dural septa is a space between the meningeal and periosteal layers of dura: a **dural sinus**. The dural sinuses are large, ependyma-lined, valveless veins that receive CSF via the arachnoid villi.

Septum	Sinus	Description
Falx cerebri: Found in the longitudinal fissure	Superior sagittal sinus	• Long longitudinally oriented sinus that receives most arachnoid villi (and CSF) • Lateral, blood-filled extensions called **lateral lacunae** are present • Terminates posteriorly in the **confluence of the sinuses**
	Inferior sagittal sinus	• Found in the inferior free edge of the falx cerebri • Terminates by joining the **great cerebral vein** to form the **straight sinus**
Tentorium cerebelli: Found between the occipital lobes and the cerebellum; divides cranial vault into supra- and infratentorial compartments	Straight sinus	Terminates posteriorly in the confluence of the sinuses
	Transverse sinus	• **Tentorial incisure** or **notch** permits passage of the brainstem from supra- to infratentorial regions • Begin at the confluence of the sinuses • Terminates by changing into the **sigmoid sinus,** which is continuous with the **internal jugular vein**
Falx cerebelli: Found between the cerebellar hemispheres	Occipital sinus	Terminates superiorly in the confluence of the sinuses

(continued)

Septum	Sinus	Description
Diaphragma sella: Circular diaphragm over the sellae turcica to protect the hypophysis; contains aperture for passage of hypophyseal stalk	Cavernous sinus	• Pair of sinuses on either side of the sella turcica, connected by small intercavernous sinuses • Drain posteriorly into the **superior petrosal sinus** (joins the junction of the transverse and sigmoid sinuses) and **inferior petrosal sinus** (exits the skull via the jugular foramen to join the internal jugular vein) • Wall contains: CN III, IV, V₁, and V₂ • Lumen contains internal carotid artery and CN VI

Clinical Significance

Lesions affecting the cavernous sinus (e.g., internal carotid artery rupture) may affect the nerves passing through or in the wall. Tumors of the hypophysis (pituitary gland) may compress the sinus, leading to cavernous sinus syndrome, ophthalmoplegia, and sensory loss over the superior aspect of the face.

The cavernous sinus is connected anteriorly with the facial vein through the ophthalmic veins; increased pressure in the facial vein

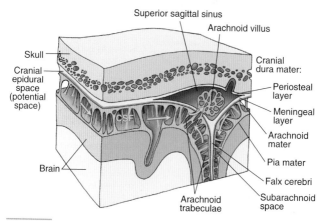

Figure 1-23. Superior sagittal sinus in frontal section.

(e.g., from a bee sting or purulent infection) may be driven into the sinus by the increased pressure.

Meninges and Spaces Around the Spinal Cord

The arrangement of the meninges is similar around the spinal cord, but there exist several differences; for example, there are no septae, and there is an epidural space.

Layer (from Outside to In)	Description	Significance
Vertebral Canal and Periosteal Covering		
Epidural space	• Fat-filled space • Location of the **internal vertebral venous plexus**	Internal vertebral venous plexus connects superiorly with the occipital sinus and basilar plexus and provides a route for the spread of infection to and from the cranial vault
Dura mater	• Tough, inflexible outer layer • Extends to S2; part inferior to the spinal cord is the **dural sac**	• Dura mater surrounding the spinal cord is continuous with the meningeal layer of dura in the cranial vault
Subdural space	Potential space	Little clinical significance
Arachnoid mater	• Delicate layer; adherent to dura by CSF pressure and **dural border cells** • Part of the **leptomeninges** with the pia mater	• Avascular • Lines the dura mater: Both extend to ~S2 vertebral level, although spinal cord ends at L1 or L2 level, creating a large **lumbar cistern**
Subarachnoid space	• CSF-filled space between the arachnoid and pia • Expanded	• Spanned by **arachnoid trabeculae**, which help stabilize the spinal cord
Pia mater	• Part of the leptomeninges with the arachnoid mater • Adherent to surface of the spinal cord	• Highly vascularized membrane • Extends below the conus medullaris as the filum terminale—internus: inside the lumbar cistern; externus: outside of the lumbar cistern connected to the coccyx • 21 pairs of lateral extensions; **denticulate ligaments** stabilize the spinal cord in the vertebral canal
Spinal Cord		

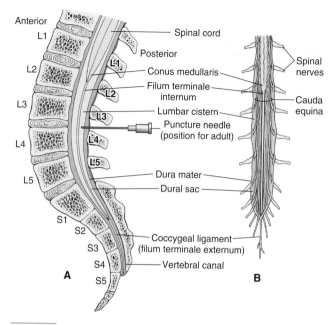

Figure 1-24. **A.** Location of spinal tap. **B.** The lumbar cistern.

Clinical Significance

The lumbar cistern, which contains CSF, nerve roots, and filum terminale, is an excellent place to remove CSF for examination (spinal tap) because there is no danger of damaging the spinal cord there (FIG. 1-24).

Anesthetic agents are injected into the spinal epidural space in a paravertebral nerve block, such as is done during childbirth.

VENTRICLES AND CEREBROSPINAL FLUID

The ventricles form as dilations of the neural tube within the brain and function as ependyma-lined, valveless veins. Each ventricle contains choroid plexus consisting of highly convoluted, vascularized epithelium that produces CSF (FIG. 1-25).

Ventricle	Significance
VENTRICLES (PRESENTED IN AN ORDER REPRESENTING THE FLOW OF CSF)	
Lateral (2)	• Located within the cerebral hemispheres • Five parts 1. Anterior (frontal) horn: Located in frontal lobe 2. Body: In frontal and parietal lobes 3. Inferior (temporal) horn: Located in temporal lobe 4. Posterior (occipital) horn: Located in parietal and occipital lobes 5. Trigone: Junction of body; posterior and inferior horns
	Interventricular Foramina (two; of Monro)
Third	Thin midline cavity located between the thalami
	Cerebral Aqueduct
Fourth	Between cerebellum and brainstem
	Lateral foramina (two; of Luschka) and Medial foramen (of Magendie)
	Subarachnoid Space

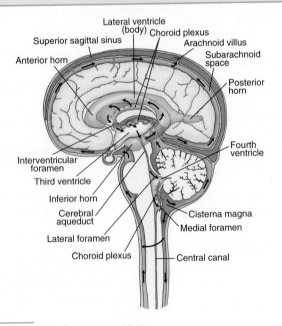

Figure 1-25. Flow of cerebrospinal fluid.

Additional Concepts

CSF a clear fluid produced by the choroid plexus at a rate of 500 to 700 mL/day. There is a total of about 150 mL in the CNS at a time. CSF provides support for the CNS, transports hormones, acts as a buffer, and removes wastes. CSF flows through the ventricular system into the subarachnoid space and into the systemic circulation at the arachnoid villi.

Clinical Significance

The trigone of the lateral ventricle contains a large tuft of choroid plexus, the **glomus**, which calcifies in adults to form a useful landmark in brain imaging.

Blockage of the interventricular foramina or cerebral aqueduct leads to hydrocephalus, or water on the brain, because CSF drainage is interrupted while production continues.

BLOOD SUPPLY

Blood supply to the brain is from two separate pairs of arteries: the vertebrals and the internal carotids.

VESSELS OF THE BRAIN		
Artery	**Origin**	**Description**
Internal carotid (2)	Common carotid	Primary supply to brain
Vertebral (2)	Subclavian	• Gives rise to basilar, posterior-inferior cerebellar, and anterior (and posterior) spinal arteries • Supply meninges, brainstem, and cerebellum
Anterior cerebral	Internal carotid	Supply medial aspect of cerebral hemispheres
Middle cerebral		Supply lateral aspect of cerebral hemispheres
Posterior cerebral	Basilar	Supply inferior aspect of cerebral hemispheres
Basilar	Vertebral	• Give rise to anterior inferior cerebellar, labyrinthine, pontine, superior cerebellar, and posterior cerebral arteries • Supply brainstem, cerebellum, and cerebrum

(continued)

Artery	Origin	Description
Anterior communicating	Anterior cerebral	Forms part of cerebral arterial circle
Posterior communicating	Joins the posterior and middle cerebral arteries	• Forms part of cerebral arterial circle • Supply cerebral peduncle, internal capsule, and thalamus
Venous drainage generally follows the arterial pattern and is indirect, draining first to the dural sinuses and then to veins.		

Additional Concepts

The **cerebral arterial circle** (of Willis) is located at the base of the brain and is the anastomosis between the vertebrobasilar and internal carotid systems (FIG. 1-26). It is formed by the posterior cerebral, posterior communicating, internal carotid, anterior cerebral, and anterior communicating arteries (FIG. 1-27).

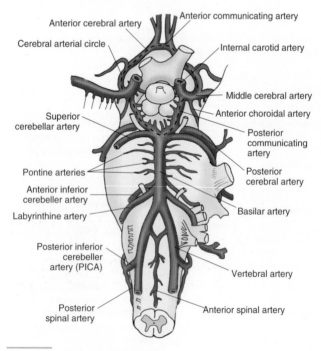

Anterior cerebral artery
Anterior communicating artery
Cerebral arterial circle
Internal carotid artery
Middle cerebral artery
Anterior choroidal artery
Superior cerebellar artery
Posterior communicating artery
Pontine arteries
Posterior cerebral artery
Anterior inferior cerebeller artery
Labyrinthine artery
Basilar artery
Posterior inferior cerebeller artery (PICA)
Vertebral artery
Posterior spinal artery
Anterior spinal artery

Figure 1-26. Arterial supply of the brain.

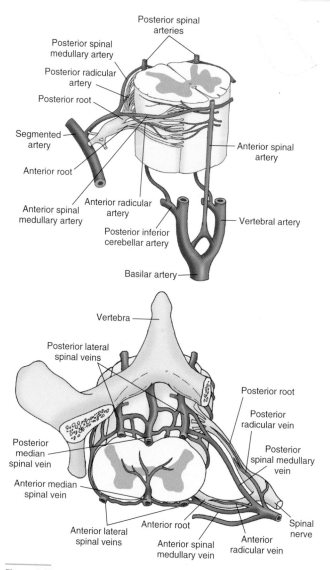

Figure 1-27. Veins of the spinal cord.

Clinical Significance

Rupture of an artery supplying the brain is a stroke (cerebrovascular accident) and typically manifests as impaired neurologic function. Occlusion may occur by an embolus (clot) blocking arterial flow. Emboli may originate locally or at some distance (the heart).

VESSELS OF THE SPINAL CORD		
Artery	**Origin**	**Description**
Vertebral	Subclavian	Give rise to anterior and posterior spinal arteries
Anterior spinal	Vertebral	Supplies anterior 2/3 of spinal cord superiorly
Posterior spinal (2)	Vertebral	Supplies posterior 1/3 of spinal cord superiorly
Segmental	Ascending cervical, deep cervical, vertebral, posterior intercostal, and lumbar	• Supply spinal cord and coverings segmentally • Anastomose with spinal arteries
Radicular: anterior and posterior	Segmental	Supply nerve roots and associated meninges
Medullary		• Variable but prevalent in the region of the cervical and lumbosacral enlargements • Supplement spinal arterial supply
Vein	**Termination**	**Description**
Anterior spinal (3)	Drained by medullary and radicular veins	• Generally parallel arterial supply • Eventually drain into the internal vertebral venous plexus
Posterior spinal (3)		
Medullary	Drain into internal vertebral venous plexus	
Radicular		
Internal vertebral venous plexus	Drain into dural sinuses of cranial vault	• Communicates with external venous plexus on external aspect of vertebrae • Potential route for infection spread from cranial vault

NEUROTRANSMITTERS

Neurotransmitters are molecules that transmit a signal from a neuron to an effector (i.e., neuron or muscle cell) across a synapse. The **synapse** is composed of the presynaptic membrane of the neuron, the synaptic cleft, and the postsynaptic membrane. They may be chemical (use neurotransmitters) or electrical, which consist of gap junctions.

COMMON CENTRAL NERVOUS SYSTEM NEUROTRANSMITTERS		
Category	Neurotransmitter	Effect
Amino acids	Glutamate	Excitatory
	GABA and glycine	Inhibitory
Biogenic amines	Dopamine	Excitatory (D1 receptors)
		Inhibitory (D2 receptors)
	Norepinephrine and epinephrine	Excitatory
	Serotonin	Excitatory or inhibitory
Purines	Adenosine triphosphate (ATP)	Excitatory or modulatory
Neuropeptides	Substance P	Excitatory
	Opioids	Inhibitory
	Acetylcholine	Excitatory

Additional Concepts

Glutamate is the most common excitatory neurotransmitter in the CNS; GABA and glycine are the most common inhibitory neurotransmitters.

Acetylcholine is used by the autonomic nervous system and at the neuromuscular junction.

IMAGING ATLAS

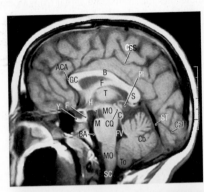

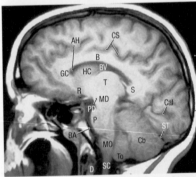

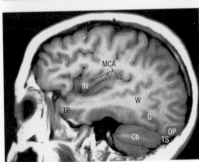

ACA	Anterior cerebral artery
AH	Anterior horn of lateral ventricle
B	Body of corpus callosum
BA	Basilar artery
BV	Body of lateral ventricle
C	Colliculi
Cal	Calcarine sulcus
Cb	Cerebellum
CQ	Cerebral aqueduct
CS	Cingulate sulcus
D	Dens (odontoid process)
F	Fornix
FV	Fourth ventricle
G	Cerebral cortex (gray matter)
GC	Genus of corpus callosum
H	Hypothalamus
HC	Head of caudate nucleus
I	Infundibulum
IN	Insular cortex
M	Mammillary body
MCA	Middle cerebral artery
MD	Midbrain
OP	Occipital pole
P	Pons
PD	Cerebral peduncle
PI	Pineal gland
R	Rostrum of corpus callosum
S	Splenium of corpus callosum
SC	Spinal cord
ST	Straight sinus
T	Thalamus
To	Cerebellar tonsil
TP	Temporal pole
TS	Transverse sinus
W	White matter
Y	Hypophysis

Sagittal Sections

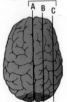

Figure 1-28. Sagittal magnetic resonance images through the brain.

Sensory System | 2

BODY

The somatosensory system consists of peripheral receptors, neural pathways, and parts of the brain involved in sensory perception.

Types of Somatosensation
- Pain and temperature
- Touch: Fine and crude
- Vibratory sense
- Proprioception: Conscious and unconscious (reflex)

Three-Neuron Chain

The somatosensory system uses a three-neuron chain (with some exceptions) to convey information from the periphery to the cerebral cortex for interpretation and processing.

Neuron	Cell Body Location	Functions
First order	Spinal ganglia or sensory ganglia of the head	Conveys sensation from periphery to the CNS
Second order	Within the central nervous system (CNS); spinal cord gray matter or brainstem	Typically gives rise to fibers that cross the midline to reach thalamus
Third order	Within the thalamus	Conveys sensation from the thalamus to the cerebral cortex

Additional Concepts

The chain of ascending neurons sends axon collaterals to mediate reflexes and affects other ascending and descending systems, an important concept for pain modulation.

The Anterolateral System

Pain, temperature, and crude touch all ascend the spinal cord as part of the **anterolateral system** located in the anterior aspect of the **lateral funiculus** and lateral aspect of the **anterior funiculus** (FIG. 2-1).

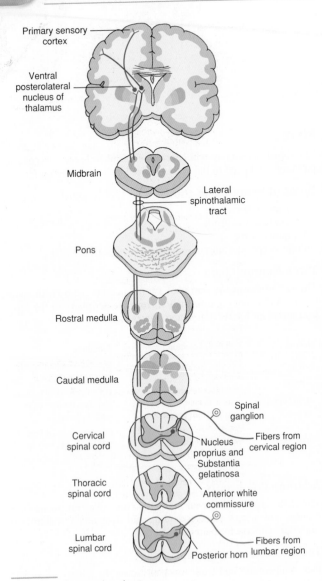

Figure 2-1. The anterolateral system.

Sense/Tract	Description	Functions
Pain and temperature/ lateral spino- thalamic	• Peripheral processes of first-order neurons end as free nerve endings; central processes enter **posterolateral tract** (of Lissauer); synapse on second-order neurons in posterior horn of spinal cord, including the **substantia gelatinosa** and **nucleus proprius**. • Second-order neurons decussate via the **anterior white commissure** and ascend as the lateral spinothalamic tract; send axon collaterals to brainstem **reticular formation**; terminate in ventral posterolateral (VPL) nucleus of thalamus. • Third-order neurons in the VPL of the thalamus project to the postcentral gyrus: primary sensory cortex (areas 3, 1, 2) via the posterior limb of **internal capsule**.	• Mediate pain, temperature, and itch • Somatotopically organized • Important in the localization of stimuli • Reach consciousness
Crude touch/ anterior spino- thalamic	• Peripheral processes of first-order neurons end as free nerve endings and on Merkel disks; central processes synapse on second-order neurons in posterior horn of spinal cord. • Second-order neurons decussate via the anterior white commissure and ascend as the anterior spinothalamic tract; send axon collaterals to brainstem reticular formation; terminate in VPL of thalamus. • Third-order neurons in the VPL of the thalamus project to the postcentral gyrus: primary sensory cortex (areas 3, 1, 2) via the posterior limb of internal capsule.	• Mediate light touch • Reach consciousness
Pain, temperature and touch/ spinoreticular	• Cell bodies within the CNS are found in the intermediate gray and anterior and posterior horns. • Project to multiple synaptic contacts within the brainstem reticular formation • Much of the tract is composed axon collaterals from spinothalamic fibers.	Involved in adjusting the level of attention to incoming sensation

(continued)

Sense/Tract	Description	Functions
Pain/spinohy-pothalamic	• Cell bodies within the CNS are found in the intermediate gray and anterior and posterior horns. • Project to widespread hypothalamic nuclei	Influence the autonomic response to incoming pain
Pain, temperature and touch/spinotectal	• Fibers that are part of the anterolateral system terminate in the **superior** and **inferior colliculi**.	Influence reflexive head movement
Pain/spino-mesencephalic	• Fibers arise from cells in the posterior horn and ascend as part of the anterolateral system.	Influence descending pain control mechanisms

Descending Pain Control Mechanisms

Descending pain control mechanisms are composed of various descending pathways that serve to inhibit ascending pain information. The most commonly accepted theory is the **gate control** theory of pain. The theory indicates that at each point in the ascending pain pathway, it is possible for a descending fiber to inhibit the ascending pain signal (i.e., act as a "gate" for the transmission). Such points include local inhibition in the spinal cord, brainstem reticular formation, and thalamus.

Additional Concepts

The primary sensory cortex has a somatotopic organization, which is represented by the homunculus: a representation of the body superimposed on the primary sensory cortex that indicates disproportionate representation of some body parts over others (e.g., the hand versus the back) (Fig. 2-2).

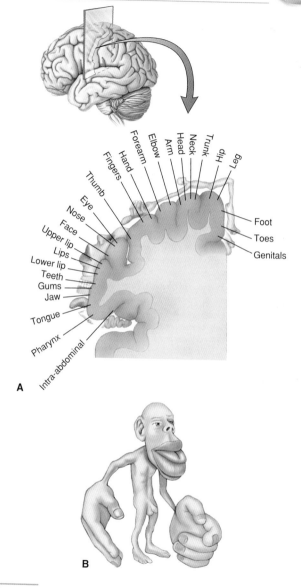

Figure 2-2. **A.** A somatotopic map of the body surface onto primary somatosensory cortex. **B.** Somatosensory homunculus.

Cerebellar Tracts for the Body

Information enters the cerebellum from the spinal cord and brainstem, which the cerebellum uses to coordinate movements. The information includes touch, pressure, and unconscious proprioception from muscle spindles and Golgi tendon organs.

Tract	Description	Functions
Anterior spinocerebellar (Fig. 2-3)	• Peripheral processes of first-order neurons end on **Golgi tendon organs** and **muscle spindles**; central processes enter posterior root to synapse on **spinal border cells** around the anterior horn between L1 and S2 cord levels. • Second-order neurons give rise to fibers that decussate in the anterior white commissure and ascend in the lateral funiculus as the **anterior spinocerebellar tract**; fibers decussate (back to the side of origin) as they enter the cerebellum via the **superior cerebellar peduncle**. • Fibers ascend to cerebellar cortex as **mossy fibers**.	• Unconscious proprioceptive information for control of groups of muscles and coordination of the lower limbs • Act as afferent limb of stretch reflexes
Posterior spinocerebellar (Fig. 2-4A)	• Peripheral processes of first-order neurons end on Golgi tendon organs and muscle spindles primarily in lower limbs; central processes enter posterior root to synapse on second-order neurons in the **posterior thoracic nucleus**. • Second-order neurons are located in the posterior thoracic nucleus, only found between the C8 and L3 cord levels; ascending processes ascend in the ipsilateral lateral funiculus as the **posterior spinocerebellar tract** and enter the cerebellum via the **inferior cerebellar** peduncle. • Fibers ascend to cerebellar cortex as mossy fibers.	• Unconscious proprioceptive information for fine coordination and control of individual muscles • Act as afferent limb of stretch reflexes
Cuneocerebellar (Fig. 2-4B)	• Peripheral processes of first-order neurons end on Golgi tendon organs and muscle spindles, primarily in upper limbs; central processes enter fasciculus cuneatus to ascend to synapse in the medulla on the **accessory (lateral) cuneate nucleus**. • Second-order neurons are located in the accessory cuneate nucleus; give rise to fibers that enter the ipsilateral cerebellum via the inferior cerebellar peduncle.	• Posterior spinocerebellar (lower limb) and Cuneocerebellar (upper limb) tracts are homologs

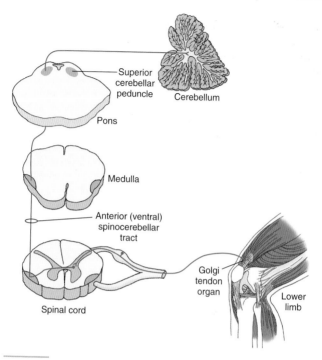

Figure 2-3. Anterior spinocerebellar tract.

The posterior thoracic nucleus is also known by its eponym, the **dorsal nucleus (of Clarke)**.

Additional Concepts

Interestingly, there is not a well-defined homolog to the anterior spinocerebellar tract for the upper limb. This is likely because we do relatively little working of the upper limb musculature in "groups," such as is done when standing or walking.

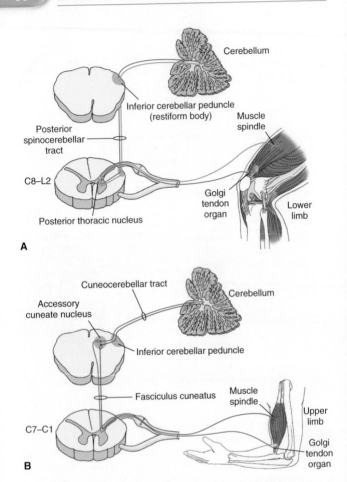

Figure 2-4. **A.** Posterior spinocerebellar tract. **B.** Cuneocerebellar tract.

Posterior Columns

Tract	Description	Functions
Posterior columns (Fig. 2-5)	• Peripheral processes of first-order neurons innervate **Pacinian corpuscles, Meissner corpuscles**, Golgi tendon organs, and muscle spindles; central processes from the lower limb arrange themselves somatotopically and ascend as the **fasciculus gracilis**, those from the upper limb form the **fasciculus cuneatus**; terminate on second-order cells in the nucleus gracilis and cuneatus in the medulla. • Processes from second-order neurons cross the midline as **internal arcuate fibers** at the level of the **sensory decussation** in the caudal medulla; the crossed fibers arrange themselves somatotopically to form the **medial lemniscus**, the medial lemniscus terminates in the VPL of the thalamus. • Third-order neurons in the VPL of the thalamus project to the postcentral gyrus: primary sensory cortex (areas 3, 1, 2) via the posterior limb of internal capsule.	• Convey information on fine touch, conscious proprioception, and vibratory sense

Additional Concepts

Unlike other sensory systems, the posterior column pathways do not send axon collaterals to the brainstem reticular formation as they project cranially. The information ascending regarding fine touch does not reflexively initiate a pain control mechanism, nor do they need to "activate" the cortex.

HEAD

Trigeminal Sensory System

The trigeminal sensory system is responsible for all of the various sensory modalities for the face and much of the head, excluding special senses (Fig. 2-6).

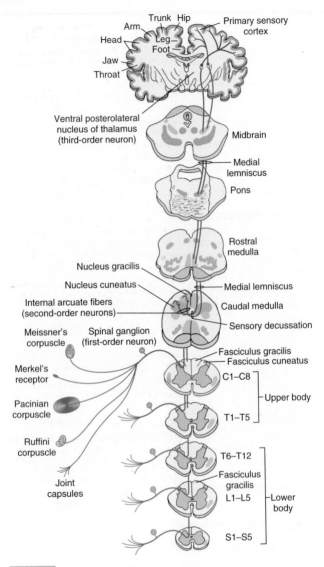

Figure 2-5. Posterior column medial lemniscus pathway.

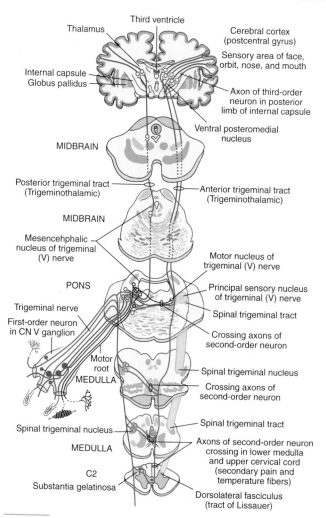

Figure 2-6. Trigeminal sensory system.

Sense/Structure	Description	Functions
Pain and temperature and touch/spinal trigeminal tract and nucleus	• Peripheral processes of first-order neurons end as free nerve endings or contact Merkel disks; first-order cell bodies are in the trigeminal, geniculate, glossopharyngeal, or vagal ganglia; central processes enter the brainstem via the trigeminal (CN V), facial (CN VII), glossopharyngeal (CN IX), or vagus (CN X) nerves; fibers ascend or descend via the **spinal trigeminal tract** to synapse on second-order neurons of the **spinal trigeminal nucleus** (C_3-midpons) located immediately medial to the tract. • Second-order fibers cross the midline to ascend to the VPM of the thalamus as the **anterior trigeminothalamic tract**; fibers also send axon collaterals to the brainstem reticular formation. • Third-order neurons in the VPL of the thalamus project to the postcentral gyrus: primary sensory cortex (areas 3, 1, 2) via the posterior limb of internal capsule.	• The spinal trigeminal tract is a homolog of the posterolateral tract • The spinal trigeminal tract allows first-order central processes to ascend or descend: pain, caudal 1/3; touch, cranial 2/3
Fine touch, conscious proprioception and vibratory sense/trigeminal ganglion	• Peripheral processes of first-order neurons innervate Pacinian and Meissner corpuscles; first-order cell bodies are in the trigeminal, geniculate, glossopharyngeal, or vagal ganglia; central processes terminate on second-order neurons in the **principal sensory nucleus**. • Second-order fibers cross the midline to ascend as part of the anterior trigeminothalamic tract to the VPM of the thalamus; fibers from the oral region travel bilaterally; those travelling ipsilaterally form the small **posterior trigeminothalamic tract** to terminate in the ipsilateral thalamus. • Third-order neurons in the VPL of the thalamus project to the postcentral gyrus: primary sensory cortex (areas 3, 1, 2) via the posterior limb of internal capsule.	• Functions similarly to the posterior columns of the spinal cord • The principal sensory nucleus is also known as the **chief sensory nucleus**

(continued)

Sense/Structure	Description	Functions
Unconscious proprioception/mesencephalic tract and nucleus	• Peripheral fibers of cells in the **mesencephalic nucleus** innervate muscles spindles and Golgi tendon organs. • Central processes project to the cerebellum and innervate the **trigeminal motor nucleus** to mediate reflexes and chewing.	Mediates unconscious or reflex proprioception from the temporomandibular joint, periodontal ligaments, and facial musculature

Additional Concepts

The trigeminal ganglion is homologous to a spinal ganglion, containing pseudounipolar primary afferents. It is also known as the **semilunar** or **Gasserian ganglion.**

CN V, CN VII, IX, and X contribute sensory fibers to the ear, middle ear cavity (CN IX), and external ear (CNs V, IX, and X).

The mesencephalic nucleus is the only population of pseudounipolar, first-order cell bodies in the CNS. It is important in the jaw-jerk reflex and used by humans primarily as infants for suckling.

Motor System | 3

PYRAMIDAL SYSTEM

The voluntary motor system is composed of white matter tracts descending from the brain to the periphery. It typically involves a two-neuron chain: an upper motor neuron (UMN) that is located in the central nervous system (CNS) and a lower motor neuron (LMN) that stimulates effectors in the periphery (Fig. 3-1).

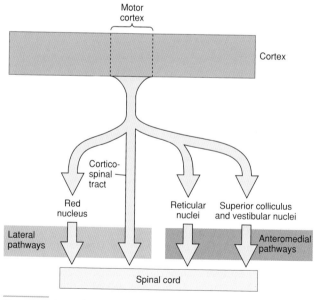

Figure 3-1. Descending motor control.

PYRAMIDAL SYSTEM: VOLUNTARY PATHWAYS

Tract	Description	Function
Anterior corticospinal Axial body	• UMN located in primary motor cortex, precentral gyrus: Brodmann's area 4; UMN receives input from association and premotor cortex and motor-related thalamic nuclei • UMN fibers descend via **internal capsule** • 90% of corticospinal fibers decussate in the pyramidal decussation, the remaining 10% cross in the spinal cord at the level of the LMN they innervate	• Controls axial musculature • Most fibers decussate in the spinal cord (anterior white commissure) • Terminate on LMN in **medial intermediate zone** at all levels of the spinal cord
Lateral corticospinal Distal body		• Controls distal musculature • Fibers decussate in the caudal medulla at the pyramidal decussation • Terminate on LMN in anterior horn at all spinal cord levels • Axon collaterals that project to basal nuclei, thalamus, and reticular formation are responsible for motor overlap • Somatotopically organized
Corticonuclear (corticobulbar) Head and face	UMNs descend bilaterally, although the majority of the fibers project to the contralateral LMN target	• UMNs synapse in the brainstem (and cervical cord) on LMN nuclei associated with cranial nerves (CNs): III, IV, V, VI, VII, IX, X, XI, and XII • Bilateral control*

*The exception to bilateral control is that innervation of the facial motor nucleus is contralateral only for the lower aspect of the face; the upper parts of the nucleus that control the upper aspect of the face are innervated bilaterally.

Additional Concepts

The primary motor cortex has a somatotopic organization, which is represented by the homunculus: a representation of the body superimposed on the primary motor cortex, which indicates the disproportionate representation of some body parts over others (e.g., the hand versus the back) (FIG. 3-2).

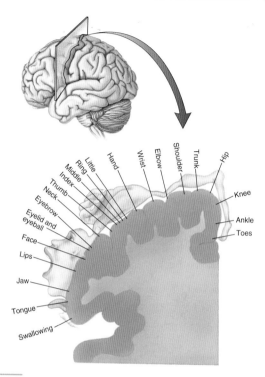

Figure 3-2. Motor homunculus.

EXTRAPYRAMIDAL SYSTEM

EXTRAPYRAMIDAL SYSTEM: INVOLUNTARY PATHWAYS (FIG. 3-3)		
Tract	**Description**	**Function**
Tectospinal	• UMN located in midbrain tectum; superior and inferior **colliculi** • Fibers descend to contralateral anterior funiculus via anteromedial aspect of spinal cord white matter • Terminate on LMNs in cervical spinal cord	• Transmits impulses for reflexive turning of the head in response to visual and auditory stimuli • Fibers cross midline in tegmental decussation, resulting in primarily contralateral control

	EXTRAPYRAMIDAL SYSTEM: INVOLUNTARY PATHWAYS (continued)	
Tract	**Description**	**Function**
Reticulospinal: Pontine and medullary	• UMN in brainstem reticular formation; pons and medulla • Pontine fibers ipsilateral • Medullary fibers bilateral	• Project to all spinal cord levels • Unconscious control of head, neck, and body
Vestibulospinal: Medial and lateral	• UMN in lateral vestibular nucleus of pons and medial vestibular nucleus of medulla • Receive input from mechanoreceptors of inner ear • Lateral vestibulospinal pathway is ipsilateral; medial pathway is bilateral • Both pathways descend anteromedial cord	• Lateral vestibulospinals synapse on LMN at all cord levels • Medial vestibulospinals travel through medial longitudinal fasciculus to synapse on LMNs in medial aspect of cervical cord • Both pathways are involved in head movement and the maintenance of posture

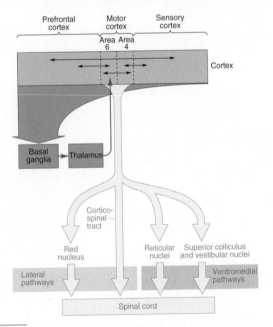

Figure 3-3. Extrapyramidal motor system.

Basal Nuclei (Ganglia)

A collection of subcortical nuclei involved in stereotyped and voluntary motor activity, the basal nuclei are the "chief" control system of the extrapyramidal motor system (FIG. 3-4). There are generally two

Structure	Description	Function
Striatum	• Caudate + Putamen = Striatum • Receives input from all regions of cerebrum and from thalamus • Output to globus pallidus and substantial nigra	• Striatum activity inhibits activity of globus pallidus and substantia nigra • Influences pyramidal system through indirect connections
Globus pallidus	• Forms medial-most part of lentiform nucleus (putamen forms lateral aspect) • Divided into external and internal parts by lamina medullaris • Receives input from striatum and subthalamic nucleus • External part projects to subthalamic nucleus via subthalamic fasciculus • Internal part projects to thalamus via thalamic fasciculus (lenticular fasciculus and ansa lenticularis)	Primary output from the basal nuclei
Substantial nigra*	• Divided into a pars compacta and pars reticulata; pars compacta composed of cells pigmented with melanin • Both parts have reciprocal connections with striatum via striatonigral and nigrostriatal tracts • Pars reticulata projects to thalamus	• Loss of dopaminergic neurons of pars compacta causes movement disorders; dopamine regulates activity through basal nuclei • Dopamine from the substantia nigra has an excitatory influence on the D_1 receptors in the striatum, which facilitates the direct pathway, while dopamine inhibits the D_2 receptor, thus inhibiting activity through the indirect pathway
Subthalamic nucleus*	• Part of diencephalon • Receives inhibitory influence input from globus pallidus • Projects excitatory input to the internal segment of the globus pallidus	Regulates activity through basal nuclei

*Groups of cells functionally associated with the basal nuclei.

pathways through the basal ganglia (FIG. 1-5) a movement activator—the direct pathway, and a movement inhibitor—the indirect pathway. The basal nuclei have no direct projection to the spinal cord; rather, they exert their influence indirectly.

Clinical Significance

Loss of dopaminergic cells in the substantia nigra pars compacta is involved in both Parkinson and Huntington disease.

Damage to the subthalamic nucleus results in ballismus, which is a violent flailing of the limbs. Damage to the striatum leads to bilateral, large-scale, ongoing uncontrolled movements primarily seen in the limbs called choreas.

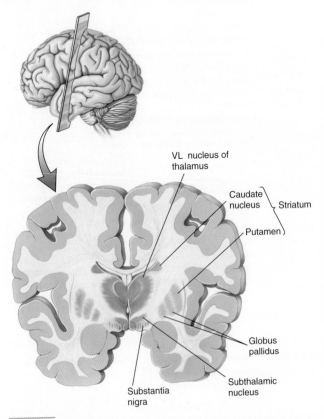

Figure 3-4. The basal nuclei.

AUTONOMIC NERVOUS SYSTEM

The nervous system can be divided into a somatic and an autonomic nervous system (ANS); the autonomic or visceral efferent system controls involuntary muscle—smooth and cardiac—and glands throughout the body. Autonomic activity is controlled by the hypothalamus, which is responsible for integrating the ANS and the endocrine system to maintain homeostasis. The ANS is divided into a sympathetic and parasympathetic division (FIG. 3-5). The preganglionic cell body is located in the CNS, and the postganglionic cell body is located in a peripheral ganglion for both systems.

Division	Description	Function
Sympathetic	• Known as thoracolumbar division owing to location of preganglionic cell bodies • Preganglionic neurons use acetylcholine as their neurotransmitter; postganglionics use norepinephrine • Preganglionic cell bodies located in **intermediolateral cell column** (T1–L2), project via **white rami communicantes** to **sympathetic trunk** or **paravertebral ganglia** or via **thoracic, lumbar,** or **sacral splanchnic nerves** to **prevertebral ganglia** found within the **aortic plexus**	• Responsible for control of stressed state: fight or flight • Results in large energy expenditure • Affects large number of structures: (1) dilator pupillae: dilates pupil; (2) salivary glands: increased viscosity of saliva and decreased blood flow to the salivary glands resulting in less saliva; (3) heart: accelerates rate and force; (4) blood vessels: vasoconstricts; (5) bronchioles: bronchodilates; (6) digestive tract: inhibits motility; (7) reproductive system: ejaculation; and (8) urinary system: activation
Parasympathetic	• Known as craniosacral division owing to location of preganglionic cell bodies • Cranial division preganglionic cell bodies located in brainstem, associated with CNs: 1. III: Preganglionic nucleus: **accessory oculomotor** (Edinger-Westphal); postganglionic cell bodies located in **ciliary** ganglion	• Responsible for control of the resting state; rest and repose

(continued)

Division	Description	Function
Parasympathetic	2. VII: Preganglionic nucleus: **superior salivatory;** postganglionic cell bodies located in **pterygopalatine** and **submandibular** ganglia 3. IX: Preganglionic nucleus: **inferior salivatory;** postganglionic cell bodies located in **otic** ganglion 4. X: Preganglionic nucleus: **dorsal motor nucleus of vagus;** postganglionic cell bodies located in wall of target organ in thorax and abdomen; supplies parasympathetic innervation up to the midtransverse colon • Sacral division preganglionic cell bodies located in sacral spinal cord S2–S4, supplies parasympathetic innervation distal to the midtransverse colon and to organs of pelvis; preganglionic fibers travel in **pelvic splanchnic nerves** to intramural ganglia in wall of target organ • Pre- and postganglionic cell bodies use **acetylcholine** as their neurotransmitter	• Responsible for energy conservation; reduces heart rate, increases digestion • CN III: Constriction of pupil and accommodation • CN VII: Lacrimation, increased oral and nasal mucosa secretion, increased saliva • CN IX: Increased saliva • CN X: Increases gastric motility and secretion, slows heart rate, and causes bronchoconstriction • Sacral parasympathetics: Lead to erection, urination, and an increase in gastric motility and secretion

Additional Concepts

Because the parasympathetic system is the energy conservation side of the ANS, it typically exerts more influence over systems than the sympathetic system, although they work in tandem at all times. The postganglionic parasympathetic fibers are very short in the parasympathetic system. In true energy-saving fashion, they are able to activate discreet muscle groups; postganglionic sympathetic fibers are relatively long, leading to massive and often not-situation-appropriate reactions to an emergency.

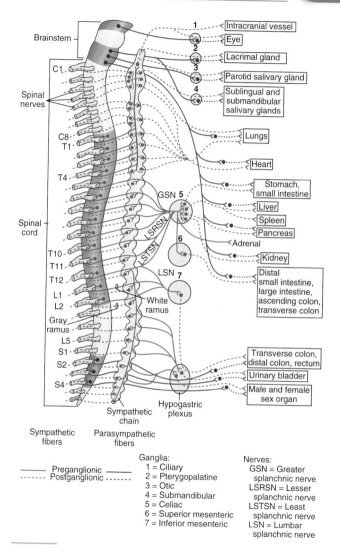

Figure 3-5. The autonomic nervous system. (Red, thoracolumbar division; blue, craniosacral division; C, cervical; L, lumbar; S, sacral; T, thoracic.)

Clinical Significance

Dysautonomia is a general term used to describe malfunction of the ANS. It may involve problems with the function of any of the multitude of structures innervated by the ANS.

CEREBELLUM

The cerebellum coordinates complex motor movements and is involved in motor learning and skilled planned motor activity. It does not initiate motor activity; rather, it controls or influences the strength, timing, and accuracy of ongoing motor activity.

It is located in infratentorially in the posterior cranial fossa.

Cerebellar Peduncles

The cerebellum is connected to the brainstem by three cerebellar peduncles (FIG. 3-6).

Peduncle	Description	Function
Superior	• Connects cerebellum to caudal midbrain and pons • Contains **dentatorubrothalamic, anterior spinocerebellar**, and **trigeminocerebellar tracts**	Major outflow pathway from cerebellum
Middle	• Connects cerebellum to pons • Contains **pontocerebellar fibers**	Major input pathway to cerebellum
Inferior	• Connects cerebellum to rostral medulla • Two parts: (1) **restiform body** containing **posterior spinocerebellar tract, cuneocerebellar tract** and **olivocerebellar tract** and (2) **juxtarestiform body** containing **vestibulocerebellar fibers** and **cerebellovestibular fibers**	Mixture of cerebellar afferents and efferents, mostly input from the spinal cord

Cerebellar Morphology

The cerebellum can be divided anterior to posterior and medial to lateral (see Chapter 1).

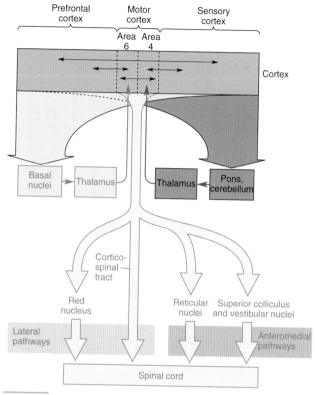

Figure 3-6. Circuitry of the cerebellar cortex.

Cerebellar Cortex

From outside to in, the cerebellar cortex is divided into a molecular layer, Purkinje cell layer, and a granule cell layer (FIG. 3-7).

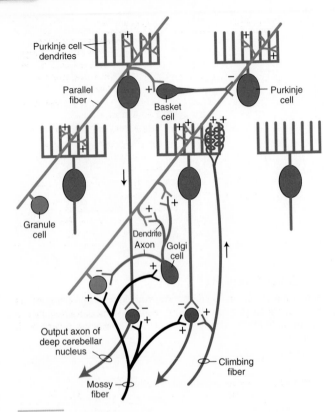

Figure 3-7. The cerebellar cortex.

Layer	Description	Function
Molecular	• Contains Purkinje cell dendritic tree • Contains parallel fibers of granule cells • Contains stellate and basket cells	Site of granule cell excitatory synapse on Purkinje cell

(continued)

Layer	Description	Function
Purkinje cell	Contains Purkinje cell bodies	• Purkinje cells represent the only outflow from the cerebellar cortex, always inhibitory (release γ-aminobutyric acid [GABA]); project to deep cerebellar nuclei and vestibular nuclei • Excited by parallel and **climbing fibers** from olivocerebellar tract • Inhibited by basket and stellate cells
Granule cell	Contains granule and Golgi cells	• Granule cells excite (glutamate) Purkinje, basket, stellate, and Golgi cells • Granule cells are inhibited by Golgi cells • Granule cells are excited by **mossy fibers** (excitatory fibers from spino- and pontocerebellar tracts)

Functional Cerebellum

Functionally, the cerebellum can be divided in terms of its involvement in primitive to more advanced movements; such a system includes the deep cerebellar nuclei associated with each division.

Anatomical Lobe	Phylogenetic Division	Functional Division	Deep Nucleus	Function
Anterior	Paleocerebellum	Spinal cerebellum	Interposed (globose + emboliform)	Locomotion: Walking, running
Primary Fissure				
Posterior	Neocerebellum	Cerebral cerebellum	Dentate	Fine movement: Playing piano, writing
Posterolateral Fissure				
Flocculonodular	Archicerebellum	Vestibular cerebellum	Fastigial	Balance: sitting upright

PHYLOGENETIC DIVISIONS

Division	Description	Function
Vestibulocerebellum	• Also known as archicerebellum • Pathway begins in inner ear; travels on CN VIII to vestibular nuclei in pons, fastigial nucleus, and flocculonodular lobe • Flocculonodular lobe also receives input from superior colliculus (visual information) and striate cortex (visual); projects back out to vestibular nuclei	• Posture, balance and equilibrium, and eye movements • Allows cerebellum to coordinate eye movements with head movement and position to keep images focused on retina
Spinocerebellum	• Also known as paleocerebellum • Receives input from spinal cord and inner ear; also from mesencephalic nucleus and cuneocerebellar fibers (upper limb) to the interposed nuclei (globose and emboliform)	• Posture, muscle tone, timing, and accuracy of ongoing movements, particularly in the trunk and limb girdles • Reciprocal connections with spinal cord allows cerebellum to influence descending spinal cord control mechanisms
Neocerebellum	• Also known as pontocerebellum • Receives both motor and sensory information from cerebral cortex • Information from cortex relays in pons (pontocerebellar fibers) • Dentatorubrothalamic tract projects back out to the **red nucleus** and thalamus	• Skilled, learned movements; hand–eye coordination with appropriate strength, timing, and precision • Cerebellum to red nucleus allows influence over all descending cortical fibers to influence volitional movements

Additional Concepts

The red nucleus projects to the inferior olivary nucleus via the central tegmental tract, which projects back to the cerebellum, forming a loop or closed circuit. Such cerebellar "circuits," whereby the cerebellar circuit is connected to the descending pathway, allow for the cerebellum to influence the descending pathway based on incoming information from the spinal cord, visual system, and inner ear.

Clinical Significance

Lesions of the flocculonodular lobe or archicerebellar lesions lead to truncal disequilibrium; gait and the trunk are affected. This causes a person to walk on a wide-base, with the trunk swaying when walking. Individuals are unsteady when standing, tend to stagger, and may appear drunk. Possible causes are a cerebellopontine angle tumor or lateral medullary syndrome (i.e., blockage of the posterior inferior cerebellar artery).

Lesions of the anterior lobe or paleocerebellum lesions are often related to alcoholism or malnutrition. The symptoms appear as gross deficits, mainly affecting the trunk and legs. The most prominent signs include dystaxia (ataxia)—poor coordination of muscles of gait and stance that cause the legs to be uncoordinated—and dystaxia (ataxia) of the trunk, causing the trunk to bob to-and-fro when walking.

Lesions of the neocerebellum or lateral hemisphere are often unilateral and may combine with anterior lobe and vermal symptoms. Lesions of the cerebellar hemispheres, dentate nucleus (anterior inferior cerebellar artery), or superior cerebellar peduncle (dentatorubrothalamic tract) may also affect speech and eye movement. Symptoms are most obvious in the upper extremity in rapid, fine movements.

Limbic System 4

THE LIMBIC SYSTEM

The limbic system is a collection of structures deep in the brain that are collectively involved in emotional memory, behavior, and memory consolidation (Fig. 4-1). The structures of the limbic system may be grouped into the medial and basal forebrain, medial temporal lobe, and limbic lobe. The limbic system activities are expressed through the hypothalamus.

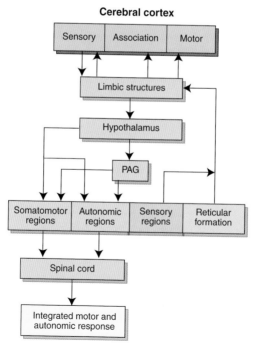

Cerebral cortex

Figure 4-1. Information flow to and from the limbic system. (PAG, periaqueductal gray.)

Group	Parts	Description	Function
Medial and basal forebrain	Septal area	• Located close to the midline and inferior to the **corpus callosum** on the medial aspect of the frontal lobe • Connections: 1. Hippocampal formation via the fornix 2. Hypothalamus via the medial forebrain bundle 3. Habenula via the stria medullaris 4. Cerebral cortex via diffuse projections	Involved in the regulation of appropriate attention to stimuli and of motivation, stimulation results in feelings of pleasure
	Ventral forebrain	• General region at base of frontal lobe deep to septal area cortex and below anterior commissure • Connections: 1. Cerebral cortex 2. Thalamus 3. Substantia nigra 4. Cingulate gyrus 5. Limbic system 6. Parahippocampal gyrus	Regulates body posture and muscle tone that accompany behavior and emotional states, such as fear, stress, and pleasure
Medial temporal lobe: Hippocampal formation and uncus	Hippocampus: Part of hippocampal formation	• Located along medial aspect of cerebrum; borders the inferior horn of the lateral ventricle within the temporal lobe • Connections: 1. Septal area via fornix 2. Hypothalamus (including mammillary bodies) via fornix 3. Dentate gyrus 4. Subiculum 5. Parahippocampal gyrus	Functions in learning and memory, short-term memory consolidation into long-term memory, and recognition of novelty
	Dentate gyrus: Part of hippocampal formation	• Located within temporal lobe • Connections: 1. Hippocampus 2. Entorhinal cortex via fornix	

(continued)

Group	Parts	Description	Function
Limbic lobe	Cingulate gyrus	• Long, arching gyrus superior to the corpus callosum • Connections: 1. Cerebral cortex 2. Thalamus 3. Mammillary bodies 4. Hypothalamus 5. Hippocampal formation 6. Septal area 7. Amygdala 8. Brainstem	Memory formation and emotional response to stimuli; regulation of visceral responses that accompany behavior
	Parahippocampal gyrus	• Parallels and lies deep to hippocampus • Continuous posteriorly with the cingulate gyrus • Major component is **entorhinal cortex** • Connections: 1. Cerebral cortex 2. Hippocampal formation	
	Amygdala	• Located within anteromedial aspect of temporal lobe, deep to the uncus • Connections: 1. Temporal and prefrontal cerebral cortex 2. Thalamus 3. Hypothalamus 4. Septal area 5. Corpus striatum 6. Brainstem	• Regulates level of aggression in behavioral and emotional states, stimulation results in rage and anxiety • Receives typical sensory input: somatosensory, sight, smell, visceral sensation, auditory and also receives sensory input on level of comfort or anxiety (from cortical sources)

Additional Concepts

The Papez circuit (Fig. 4-2) is the first pathway described involving the limbic system properly. It includes the cingulate gyrus to the hippo-campal formation to the hypothalamus (mammillary bodies) to the anterior nucleus of the thalamus back to the cingulate gyrus.

Projections from the amygdala and hipppocampus to the striatum influence motor activity as it relates to mood and emotion.

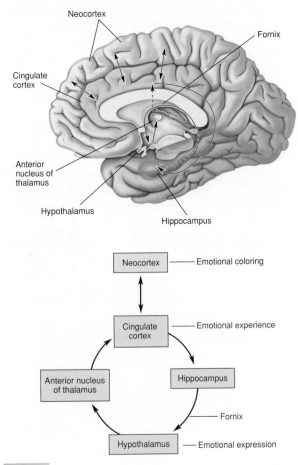

Figure 4-2. Papez circuit.

Whereas stimulation of the amygdala causes stress and anxiety, stimulation of the septal area causes pleasure and relaxation; these two systems balance control of emotional responses depending on circumstances.

The limbic system consolidates memory by **long-term potentiation**, the mechanism of memory consolidation (FIG. 4-3). One synapse fires in a particular temporal pattern, making it more likely that the synapse will be activated by the same pattern in the future. The more the synapse is activated, the more likely it will be activated in the future, allowing stimuli and responses to be paired.

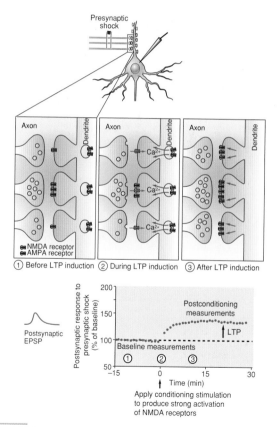

Figure 4-3. Long-term potentiation.

Clinical Considerations

The hippocampus is one of the first areas to undergo cell death in Alzheimer's disease; because it is important in consolidation of memories, individuals with Alzheimer's disease have difficulty in this area. Lesions of the amygdala result in placidity, including loss of fear, rage, and aggression. An animal with a deficit in this area is not likely to last long.

Klüver-Bucy syndrome results from bilateral destruction of the medial aspect of the temporal lobes, including the amygdala and hippocampus, resulting in placidity, hypersexuality, hyperphagia, and visual agnosia.

Korsakoff syndrome, typically a result of thiamine deficiency (often seen in people with alcoholism), leads to cell loss in the hippocampal formation and results in amnesia, confabulation, and disorientation.

Chemical Senses | 5

The chemical senses are those that involve dissolved chemicals in order to initiate impulses from receptors. The chemical senses are olfaction (smell) and gustation (taste).

OLFACTION

Olfaction is a phylogenetically old sense. Various chemicals and chemical concentrations dissolved in the nasal mucosa stimulate an array of olfactory receptors, which are interpreted by the olfactory cortex to create the sense of smell (FIG. 5-1). Our ability to detect the huge range of odors that we are capable of is still poorly understood.

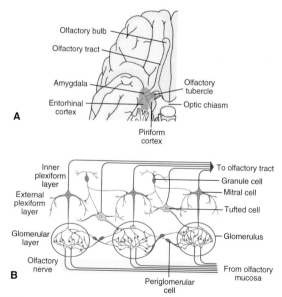

Figure 5-1. The olfactory system. **A.** Olfactory cortex. **B.** Contents of the olfactory bulb. (*continued*)

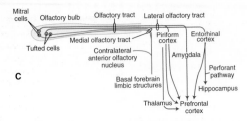

Figure 5-1. (*continued*) **C.** Central connections of the olfactory system.

Part	Description	Connections	Function
Olfactory epithelium	Three cell types: 1. **Basal:** Stem cells; give rise to olfactory receptor neurons 2. **Supporting:** Secrete granules onto mucosal surface 3. **Receptor:** First-order, bipolar neurons capable of mitosis; cilia provide transduction surface for odor stimulants	Signals are transmitted from the olfactory epithelium to the olfactory bulb by passing through the **cribriform plate** of the **ethmoid**; the fibers passing through the cribriform plate collectively form the **olfactory nerve** (CN I)	Detects and responds to odorants from the environment and relays information to the olfactory bulb
Olfactory bulb	• Site of second-order neurons: **Mitral cells** and **tufted cells** • Located on the cribriform plate of the ethmoid	• Receives input from the olfactory nerve • Conducts impulse from olfactory neurons to olfactory cortex via the **olfactory tract** and **lateral olfactory stria**	• Allows a specific response to stimulants through selective stimulation of receptors and second-order neurons
Olfactory tract	Contains **anterior olfactory nucleus**	Divides into **lateral** and **medial olfactory stria**	Anterior olfactory nucleus regulates and modulates the distribution of olfactory information

(*continued*)

Part	Description	Connections	Function
Olfactory cortex	• Site of the third-order neuron • Overlies uncus, part of the **prepiriform** and **entorhinal cortices** • Possesses a direct cortical projection (bypasses the thalamus)	Sends impulses to the dorsomedial nucleus of thalamus, basal forebrain, and limbic system	Allows for specific perception of odor through connections with limbic system: Emotional response and memory formation and retrieval related to odor

Additional Concepts

The olfactory receptor cells (neurons) are some of the only neurons in the human nervous system that are capable of mitosis.

Clinical Considerations

Fracture of the thin cribriform plate that damages the olfactory receptor cells is a common cause of anosmia (loss of smell). Puncture or tear of the dura mater is common, causing cerebrospinal fluid to leak from the nasal cavity. Smell returns after regeneration of the receptor cells.

GUSTATION (TASTE)

Taste is perceived through stimulation of the taste buds. Flavor is taste plus olfactory, somatosensory, visual, and limbic input. Mood, proximity to the previous meal, temperature, smell, and the appearance and feel of food all affect flavor.

Part	Description	Connections	Function
Gustatory receptor	• Located within taste buds of the tongue and oral cavity • Cilia extend through taste pore • Modified epithelial cells with neuron-like properties • Replaced every 1–2 weeks	Depolarized gustatory cell synapses with first-order neuron whose dendrites wrap the cell	• Cilia project through pore and are bathed by saliva; chemicals cause the cells to depolarize • Five tastants: Sweet, sour, bitter, salty, and umami (savory)

(continued)

Part	Description	Connections	Function
First-order neuron	• Pseudounipolar cells located in the **geniculate** (CN VII), **petrosal** (CN IX), and **nodose** (CN X) **ganglia** • Forms afferent limb of reflex: Coughing, swallowing • Carried on processes of CNs VII, IX, and X	• CNs convey impulses from tongue to **nucleus solitarius** via the solitary tract • Anterior 2/3 of tongue: CN VII • Posterior 1/3 of tongue: CN IX • Epiglottis, soft palate: CN X	Relays neural information from tongue to nucleus solitarius
Second-order neuron	Located in medulla in the gustatory portion (rostral-most) of nucleus solitarius: the **gustatory nucleus**	• Receives input from CNs • Fibers pass ipsilaterally via the **central tegmental tract** to the medial-most part of the **ventral posteromedial** (VPM) nucleus of the thalamus • Projects to **parabrachial nucleus** of pons	• Second-order neurons of the nucleus solitarius receive and combine taste information from all three CNs carrying taste • Parabrachial nucleus passes taste information to the hypothalamus and amygdala
Third-order neuron	Located in the medial-most part of the VPM of the thalamus	• Receive input from nucleus solitarius • Conveys taste information to cortex via internal capsule	Conveys ipsilateral taste information from VPM to gustatory cortex
Gustatory cortex	• Brodmann's area 36 • Located near insula and medial surface of frontal operculum near the base of the central sulcus	• Receives input from VPM • Projects to orbital cortex of frontal lobe and to the amygdala	Integrates taste information with other areas (limbic, olfactory, visual, and sensory systems) to produce perception of flavor

Clinical Significance

Smoking is the most common cause of ageusia (loss of taste).

Visual System | 6

The visual system is responsible for processing images formed from light hitting the retina. It is composed of neural relay systems that begin in the eye, travel in the optic nerve and tract to the lateral geniculate nucleus (LGN) of the thalamus and finally to the visual cortex.

STRUCTURES

Part	Description	Connections	Function
Eye	Composed of three layers (tunics): 1. Outer: Sclera and cornea 2. Middle: Choroid, iris, and ciliary body 3. Inner: Retina	• Retina is composed of seven layers • Impulses are conducted from superficial to deep	• Structure of the eye focuses light on the retina, particularly the center • Impulses from photoreceptors sent to ganglion cells, which form the optic nerve
Retina	• Composed of five cell types, from superficial to deep: 1. Photoreceptors 2. Bipolar cells 3. Horizontal cells 4. Amacrine cells 5. Ganglion cells • **Optic disk** (papilla): Medial to fovea, blind spot; contains axons from ganglion cells • **Macula lutea:** Yellow pigmented area surrounding **fovea centralis;** area of highest visual acuity; contains cones only	Photoreceptors are stimulated, sending an impulse that eventually stimulates ganglion cells that form the optic nerve	Receives focused images from the cornea and lens, which initiates an impulse that is transmitted to the optic nerve

Retina

The seven-layered inner tunic of the eye develops as an outgrowth of the diencephalon; it has five cell types within it (FIG. 6-1). The seven layers of the retina from superficial to deep are:

1. Retinal pigmented epithelium
2. Photoreceptor layer
3. Outer nuclear layer
4. Outer plexiform layer
5. Inner nuclear layer
6. Inner plexiform layer
7. Ganglion cell layer

Cell Type	Description	Connections	Function
Photoreceptor	• Two types: **Rods** and **cones** • Consist of cell body and synaptic terminal; respond to light • Glutamate is the neurotransmitter	Synapse on bipolar and horizontal cells	• Rods: Provide low-acuity images; monochromatic • Cones: Provide images with high visual acuity; color vision; need a lot of light • Both convert stimulation from light into neuronal impulses
Bipolar	• Receive impulse from photoreceptors • Located between inner and outer plexiform layer • Glutamate is the neurotransmitter	Terminate on ganglion cells	Provide pathway from photoreceptors to ganglion cells
Amacrine	• Located between inner nuclear layer and outer plexiform layer • γ-Aminobutyric acid (GABA), dopamine, and acetylcholine act as neurotransmitters	Synapse on ganglion cells in the outer plexiform layer	Inhibit ganglion cells

(continued)

Cell Type	Description	Connections	Function
Horizontal	• Located in the nuclear and plexiform layers • GABA is the neurotransmitter	Synapse on bipolar cells	• Modify the responses of the bipolar cells • Role in color differentiation • Responsible for lateral inhibition of photoreceptors
Ganglion	• Only source of output from retina, act as third-order afferents • Glutamate is the neurotransmitter • Axons leave retina as optic nerve (CN II)	Axons continue to optic chiasm as optic nerve	Influenced by bipolar and horizontal cells

Additional Concepts

The ganglion cells form the optic nerve (CN II); they project to the:

• Thalamus (LGN)
• **Superior colliculus:** To mediate visual reflexes and for dynamic visual map of environment
• Hypothalamus (suprachiasmatic nucleus): To mediate circadian rhythms
• Pretectal nucleus: Role in mediating behavioral responses to light: pupillary light reflex, optokinetic reflex, accommodation reflex, and circadian rhythms. **Lateral inhibition** is the property of an activated neuron to inhibit excitation of nearby neurons, thereby providing increased discrimination of the excited neuron.

PATHWAYS

Visual Pathway

The visual image is transferred from the retina to the cerebral cortex by the central visual pathway. Along the way, the image is distributed to various parts of the central nervous system (CNS).

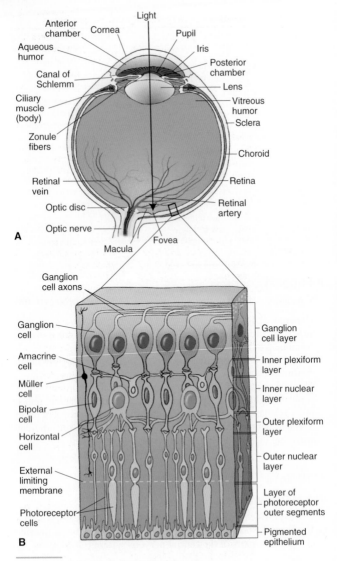

Figure 6-1. **A.** The eye. **B.** The layers of the retina.

Part	Description	Connections
Optic nerve (CN II)	• Actually a myelinated tract of the diencephalon • Invested with arachnoid, pia, and subarachnoid space	• Ganglion cell axons exit the eye at the optic disk and travel to the optic chiasm • Transmit impulses from retina to optic chiasm
Optic chiasm	• Impulses from nasal retina cross midline to join impulses from temporal retina of contralateral eye; thus, visual information from the left visual field of both eyes travels down the right side of the visual pathway and vice versa • Located immediately superior to hypophysis	Receives input from CN II; nasal retinal fibers cross and leave posteriorly as optic tract
Optic tract	Conveys matched visual field information from each eye posteriorly; has fibers from the ipsilateral temporal hemiretina and contralateral nasal hemiretina	Connects the optic chiasm to the LGN of the thalamus
Lateral geniculate nucleus	• Part of the posterior aspect of the thalamus • Composed of six layers, separated by the visual field to which they are related: • Ipsilateral temporal hemiretina (layers 2, 3, and 5) • Contralateral nasal hemiretina (layers 1, 4, and 6) • And/or identified by cell size: • Magnocellular layers (layers 1 and 2): Responsible for relaying contrast and movement information • Parvocellular layers (layers 3–6): Responsible for relaying color and form information	• Fibers travel to the occipital lobe as the geniculocalcarine tract or optic radiations • Inferior visual field fibers terminate on the superior bank of the calcarine sulcus, superior visual field fibers terminate on the inferior bank of the calcarine sulcus
Optic radiations	• Fan out as the retrolenticular part of the internal capsule • Fibers extending inferomedially into the temporal lobe are known as **Meyer's loop**	• Transmit impulses from LGN to primary occipital cortex • Left optic radiations carry all information from right visual fields of both eyes and vice versa

(continued)

Part	Description	Connections
Primary visual cortex	• Cortical area (17) along the calcarine sulcus of the occipital lobe • Visual information is inverted and reversed upon reaching area 17 • Information from the inferior visual fields terminates superior to the calcarine sulcus on the cuneate gyrus; information from superior visual fields terminates inferior to the calcarine sulcus on the lingual gyrus	• Primary visual cortex sorts and sends information to other cortical areas: Visual association cortices (18 and 19) • Possesses retinotopic organization: • Central part of retina is represented most posteriorly and occupies a disproportionately large amount of the visual cortex • More peripheral parts are represented more anteriorly

Additional Concepts

Because the optic nerve is a tract of the diencephalon, it is not actually a nerve. A retinotopic organization is maintained from the retina all of the way to the primary visual cortex.

MNEMONIC

The word **SLIM** can help you remember the relationship between elements of the visual system:

The **S**uperior Colliculus receives input from the **L**ateral Geniculate Nucleus. The **I**nferior Colliculus receives input from the **M**edial Geniculate Nucleus.

Clinical Significance

PAPILLEDEMA

The optic nerve is part of the diencephalon and as such is invested with arachnoid, pia, and subarachnoid space; increases in intercranial pressure compress the nerve, leading to papilledema (swelling of the optic disk).

VISUAL DEFICITS

Visual deficits are named for visual field loss, not retinal loss. The optic chiasm lies immediately superior to the pituitary gland; thus, a pituitary tumor may put pressure on the fibers running through the chiasm. Whereas midsagittal pressure results in bitemporal hemianopia, bilateral compression from calcification of the internal carotid arteries in the cavernous sinus may result in binasal hemianopia.

Visual Processing

Visual processing involves fast and slow conjugate eye movements. Saccades are fast, steplike movements that bring objects onto the retina. The velocity of a saccadic eye movement is too fast for the visual system to relay the information it receives, so the CNS computes the size of the movement in advance and initiates it reflexively. Smooth, slow tracking movements allow images to stay on the fovea centralis.

Action or Structure	Description	Function
Saccadic movements	• Fast, steplike movements • Initiated by the **frontal eye fields:** part of the prefrontal cortex and the **superior colliculus**	• Bring objects of interest onto retina • Velocity too great for visual system, so CNS computes size of movement in advance and suppresses perception of vision during movement
Slow pursuit movements	Slow, cortically driven tracking	Allows images to stay on the fovea centralis
Visual association cortex	• Brodmann's areas 18, 19, 20, and 37	• Provides meaning associated with vision • Projects "where" information to **parieto-occipital cortex** and projects "what" information to **occipitotemporal cortex** • Separates complex visual information into two "streams" 1. Dorsal: Where 2. Ventral: What

Additional Concepts

Nystagmus is the combined action of a fast saccadic eye movement in one direction and a slow pursuit movement in the opposite direction, which is necessary to keep objects of interest focused on the retina.

Auditory and Vestibular Systems | 7

The auditory and vestibular systems consist of morphologically and functionally interconnected structures. Both are housed in the inner ear deep in the temporal bone, both send axons centrally that travel in the vestibulocochlear nerve (CN VIII), and disruptions of one system often affect the other.

AUDITORY SYSTEM

The auditory system deals with the sense of hearing. The hearing apparatus is divided into an outer, middle, and inner ear (FIG. 7-1).

Part	Description	Function
Outer	• Consists of the auricle and external auditory meatus • Extends medially to tympanic membrane, which vibrates when sound vibrations contact it	• Funnels sound from outside world to tympanic membrane • Sensory innervation by CNs V, VII, and X • Functions in sound localization
Middle	Consists of tympanic membrane, ossicles (malleus, incus, and stapes), muscles (tensor tympani and stapedius), and auditory tube	• Movement of tympanic membrane causes the ossicles to vibrate in turn to transmit vibration to oval window, which leads to inner ear • Sensory innervation by CN IX • Muscles dampen sound; auditory tube equalizes pressure with atmospheric
Inner	• Consists of receptor organs within the cochlear duct of the membranous labyrinth • Vibrations originating at oval window stimulate hair cells in cochlear duct; part of the **Organ of Corti**	• Vibration of the footplate of the stapes in the oval window results in vibration of the basilar membrane, upon which the Organ of Corti sits; the Organ of Corti is composed of receptor cells called hair cells • Hair cells transduce vibrations into a neural signal, which is carried centrally by CN VIII

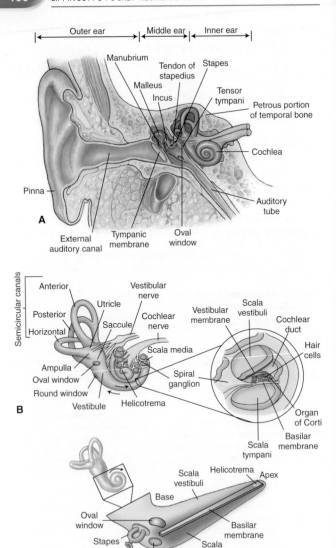

Figure 7-1. **A.** The auditory apparatus. **B.** The inner ear. **C.** The cochlea.

Additional Concepts

Three features of sounds we perceive:

1. Location: A central nervous system (CNS) comparison mediated by the superior olivary nucleus
2. Frequency: Determined by where along basilar membrane vibration is greatest
3. Amplitude: Determined by the number of hair cells that are stimulated and thereby the number of afferent nerve fibers that are firing

Clinical Significance

CONDUCTION DEAFNESS

Conduction deafness results when any part of the external or middle ear is damaged in such a way as to impede transfer of sound vibrations to the inner ear.

NERVE DEAFNESS

Nerve deafness results from damage to the cochlea, CN VIII, or central auditory pathway.

Auditory Pathway

The auditory pathway begins with the hair cells of the organ of Corti and ends in the primary auditory cortex (FIG. 7-2).

Part	Description	Function
Organ of Corti	Inner and outer hair cells are stimulated by movement of endolymph in the cochlear duct and movement of the basilar membrane	Bending of the hair cells causes depolarization, which stimulates the first-order afferents of CN VIII
Vestibulocochlear nerve (CN VIII)	• Contains primary afferent fibers of auditory system • Cell bodies located in **spiral ganglion** located along the bony **modiolus**	Transmits impulses from cochlear duct to cochlear nuclei of the brainstem

(continued)

Part	Description	Function
Cochlear nuclei	• Located in the medulla • Receive input from CN VIII • Divided into a dorsal and ventral group	• Ventral nuclei project bilaterally to superior olivary nucleus and through lateral lemniscus to contralateral inferior colliculus • Dorsal nuclei project contra-laterally to inferior colliculi via the **acoustic stria** • Crossing fibers form the trapezoid body
Superior olivary nucleus	• Located in the pons • Conveys information bilaterally to inferior colliculi • Fibers travel in lateral lemniscus	• Receives input from ventral cochlear nuclei • Projects bilaterally • Involved in sound localization by making a temporal comparison of information coming from each ear
Inferior colliculi	• Located in midbrain tectum • Receives input from dorsal and ventral cochlear nuclei	• Sends impulses to medial geniculate nucleus of thalamus • Fibers cross midline via commissure of inferior colliculus; projects to superior colliculus to mediate audiovisual reflexes
Medial geniculate nucleus	Part of thalamus	• Receives projections from inferior colliculus • Projects to auditory cortex via sublenticular part of internal capsule, the auditory radiations
Primary auditory cortex	• Located along superior temporal gyrus: Brodmann's areas 41 and 42, known as the transverse gyrus of Heschl • Tonotopic organization: Lower frequencies more anterior, higher frequencies more posterior	• Input from medial geniculate nucleus • Projects to auditory association cortex: Area 22 • Responsible for sound discrimination

Additional Concepts

Because the cochlear nuclei project bilaterally, to get deafness in one ear, the problem must occur at or proximal to the cochlear nuclei (i.e., organ of Corti, spiral ganglion, or CN VIII).

CN VIII is actually two nerves in one: a cochlear nerve and a vestibular nerve.

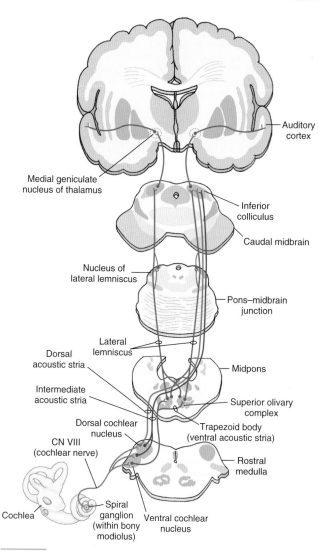

Figure 7-2. Central auditory pathway.

VESTIBULAR SYSTEM

The vestibular system is involved with the sense of equilibrium and balance. The semicircular canals are involved in detection of angular or changing movement, whereas the macular organs are involved with perceiving static position (FIG. 7-3).

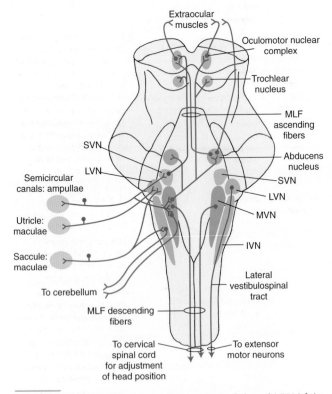

Figure 7-3. Central vestibular pathway. (SVN, superior vestibular nuclei; IVN, inferior vestibular nuclei; MVN, medial geniculate nuclei; LVN, lateral vestibular nuclei.)

Part	Description	Function
Semicircular canals	• Contain receptors for detection of angular acceleration of the head • **Cristae ampullari** located in the semicircular canals detect head movement by endolymph deformation of hair cells embedded in the gelatinous **cupula**	Deformation of the cilia of the hair cells stimulates the primary afferents of CN VIII, the cell bodies of which are located in the vestibular (Scarpa's) ganglion
Macular organs: Utricle and saccule	• Contain receptors for linear acceleration; constant • Saccule responds maximally when head is vertical • Utricle responds maximally when head is perpendicular to body • Detects position by maculae; contains otoliths within gelatinous membrane into which cilia of hair cells are embedded	• Otoliths make the gelatinous membrane "heavy," such that it responds to gravity and does not allow the gelatinous membrane to reset to resting position until head is repositioned • Deformation of the cilia of the hair cells stimulates the primary afferents of CN VIII, the cell bodies of which are located in the vestibular (Scarpa's) ganglion
Vestibular ganglion	Contains primary afferent cell bodies of CN VIII	• Projects centrally to vestibular nuclei of brainstem • Projects to cerebellum via juxtarestiform body
Vestibular nuclei	• Located in pons and rostral medulla on floor of fourth ventricle • Receive input from CN VIII, cerebellum, and contralateral vestibular nuclei • Outputs to oculomotor, abducens, and trochlear nuclei via **medial longitudinal fasciculus** • Divided into superior, inferior, medial and lateral nuclear groups	• Fibers to CN III, IV, and VI nuclei coordinate head and eye movement and mediate vestibulo-ocular reflex • Fibers synapse at cervical levels of spinal cord via medial vestibulospinal tract to control head and neck musculature • Fibers descend the length of the spinal cord via the lateral vestibulospinal tract to control balance and extensor tone • Project to cerebellum, contralateral vestibular nuclei, inferior olivary nuclei, and thalamus (ventral posterior inferior and ventral posterior lateral); project to primary vestibular cortex (area 2) and parietal lobe

Additional Concepts

The vestibulo-ocular reflex (Fig. 7-4) links the vestibular system and eye movement to keep objects of the interest in the center of the retina reflexively during head movement. The eyes move slowly opposite the direction of head movement, thus keeping the object of interest centered on the fovea centralis.

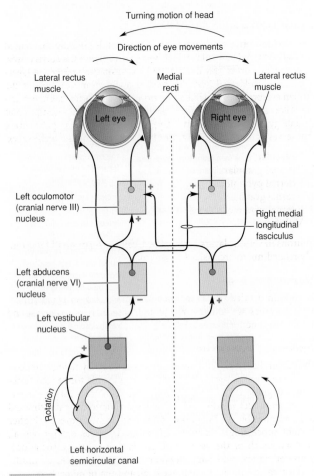

Figure 7-4. The vestibulo-ocular reflex.

Cerebral Cortex | 8

STRUCTURES AND RELATIONSHIPS

The cerebral cortex is composed of gray matter. It is highly convoluted (folded) into gyri and sulci, which serves to increase the surface area. The cerebral cortex may be classified based on the number of layers it possesses: 6 layered isocortex or neocortex composes most of the human cerebral cortex, while more primitive allocortex has fewer layers. Allocortex is divided into the archicortex of the hippocampus and dentate gyrus, which has only 3 layers and the 3–5 layers paleocortex that serves as the transitional cortex between the neo- and archicortex.

1. Molecular
2. External granular
3. External pyramidal
4. Internal granular
5. Internal pyramidal
6. Multiform

Neurons in various layers connect vertically to form small functionally related microcircuits, called *columns.*

Brodmann's Areas

Brodmann divided the cortex into 47 areas based on cytoarchitecture; the areas are still referred to today because they correspond roughly to functional areas (FIG. 8-1).

Regions of the Cortex

The cerebral cortex accomplishes complex tasks by having associative areas: areas of the cerebral cortex responsible for related functions, integration, and higher processing. Such areas may be classified as unimodal (dealing with a specific function) or multimodal (areas responsible for integrating one or more modalities for higher thought processing). Examples of unimodal areas are the visual, auditory, much of the association cortex (i.e., visual association), premotor cortex, and supplementary cortex. Examples of multimodal areas are the prefrontal, parietal, and temporal cortices.

Association areas function to produce meaning, quality, and texture to primary areas with which they are associated.

Area	Description
Sensory	• Primary somatosensory (3, 1, and 2): Postcentral gyrus; somatotopically organized as sensory homunculus; primarily involved with localization of sensation • Somatosensory association cortex (5 and 7): Superior parietal lobule; involved with adding "meaning" to sensation (e.g., rough versus smooth, heavy versus light) • Supramarginal gyrus (40): Integrates somatosensory, auditory, and visual sensation • Primary visual cortex (17): Occipital lobe; vision • Visual association cortex (18, 19, and 39): Angular gyrus; involved with adding "meaning" to visual stimuli • Primary auditory cortex (41 and 42): Superior temporal gyrus; hearing • Auditory association cortex (22): Superior temporal gyrus; language comprehension • Gustatory cortex (43): Parietal operculum and parainsular cortex; taste • Vestibular cortex (2): Postcentral gyrus; balance and equilibrium
Motor	• Primary motor cortex (4): Precentral gyrus; initiates voluntary movement • Premotor cortex (6): Anterior to precentral gyrus on the frontal lobe; prepares primary motor cortex for activity • Supplementary motor cortex (6): Frontal lobe anterior to precentral gyrus; contains program for voluntary motor movement • Frontal eye field (8): Middle frontal gyrus; eye movement
Higher function	• Prefrontal cortex (9, 10, 11, and 12): Frontal lobe; personality, motivation, future planning, primitive reflexes • Broca's speech area (44 and 45): Inferior frontal gyrus; motor aspect of speech • Wernicke's speech area (22): Superior temporal gyrus; speech comprehension

Additional Concepts

Hemispheric dominance refers to the side of the brain where language centers are located. In the majority of people, this is the left hemisphere.

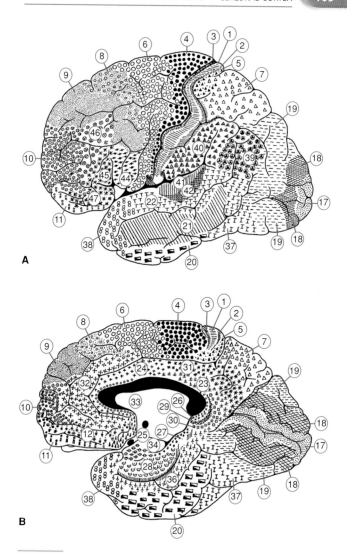

Figure 8-1. Brodmann's areas.

Note: Page numbers followed by an *f* indicate a figure.